The Holistic PCOS Guide

Natural Ways to Help Women with Polycystic Ovarian Syndrome Balance Hormones, Manage Stress, and Lose Weight Without Medication

Luna Schwartz

Table of Contents

Introduction

One in ten women of childbearing age in the world is afflicted with Polycystic Ovarian Syndrome or PCOS (Center for Disease Control and Prevention, 2019[1]). It is the most common endocrine disorder of reproductive-aged women. PCOS affects millions of people regardless of age, race, religion or culture. I have been lucky enough to win the genetic draw of being afflicted with PCOS. And from my growing up years to my adulthood, I have always struggled with this condition. Every moment, I can feel that this disorder is claiming a part of me, from my body to my mind, changing the way I feel and view the world. I always think about it because it pains me in so many levels all at the same time. This disorder has isolated me from my friends who may not be able to understand what I am going through. It has kept me away from potential partners who may be disappointed with my difficulty in bearing a child. It has isolated me from myself as I shudder to see the person facing me in the mirror. PCOS has brought out the worst in me and I know that it is the same way with other women struggling with this condition.

A large part of the difficulty with PCOS lies in the cumbersome hegemony of the scientific narrative. Yes, PCOS is a medical condition, affecting women's bodies down to the biochemical level. And most of the experts in this field are scientists, doctors and researchers who have defined PCOS and its treatment. These professionals have poured in millions of dollars in researching about how our hormones function and adapt, and how this order can be disrupted in PCOS. I have the highest admiration for these tireless heroes in the fields of research and medicine. Without them, we would not have a sophisticated understanding of PCOS and how best to treat it.

Our understanding of PCOS has become monopolized in a scientific and medical sense. Much of the research in PCOS is only appreciated in academic and scientific circles, not reaching the ordinary woman suffering from this condition. When you look at the articles and the books on PCOS, much of it is worded in scientific jargon like 'inappropriate gonadotropin secretion' or 'autosomal dominant inherited endocrine disorder'. Not only do the words sound intimidating to the ordinary person, but it also sends a signal that you need to be an expert in order to understand. There is an elitist feel to the scientific journals that try to explain PCOS. And to ordinary women struggling with this condition, it alienates us further when we have to grapple with terms we don't understand. The technical terms also make us averse to seeking the treatment we need. There is no room to question what the journals say because I felt ignorant about the condition that affects me on an everyday basis. I personally experienced this as I try to find resources in helping me understand my condition. Much of the researches online seem to have PhD graduates as an audience, and not to me living with PCOS. Books on the topic try to water it down to a much more understandable topic, but authors discuss the treatment as though it is a simple recipe book you need to follow, and all your problems will go away.

Throughout my teenage years and as I aged, I always felt insecure about my body size. Later on, I will explain some of the mechanisms of how PCOS affects your body. But one of the most prominent changes is a tendency to gain weight. Women with PCOS are more prone to gain more weight even with an ordinary diet. I know I should be proud of who I am and how I look no matter what. But society's standards of beauty made me feel I was never enough. I would see my thin peers in school running around, eating what they want and yet looked like they never put on pounds. Clothes were also a big problem for me because the clothes I liked were never in my size. I always felt like a bag of potatoes in the clothes I wore. I know I was smart, caring and friendly, but the physical body I was in did not make me feel that I was capable and good. I've tried dieting with all sorts of regiment in the market, but most programs made me really die from starvation. It was either the food was too bland for my taste or too expensive to procure. I ended up with more cheat days than actually dieting days. It is very hard to feel you are beautiful in your own skin when your self-image does not match what other people perceive is beautiful.

Mental health is also an issue that is not very much discussed when it comes to PCOS. Most of the treatment for the disorder involves hormonal injections or medications that seem to address only the physical body. But much of the pain from PCOS is derived from the mind, and not just the body. PCOS can deal a lot of damage to the emotional ego of a person that not many people are recognizing. My physical appearance of being overweight, having a lot of unwanted hair, developing acne even in my adult years and having patches of dark skin folds made me reluctant to make friends. My difficulty in getting pregnant has lowered my chances of actually finding a partner. All these body issues can trigger symptoms of depression and anxiety, as I struggled with PCOS. A combined oral contraceptive pill never did wonders for my depression, no matter how often I took it. Yes, it may relieve some symptoms, but at the end of the day, I still have to grapple with my self-image and the voices inside my head telling me all sorts of negative things. Even if my body improved with some of the medications or diet, I still thought of myself as ugly and undesirable. At my lowest point, I realized that the greatest battle I was waging was not with my body but with my mind. The most superficial area that PCOS affects is the physical body. I had to reorient myself in viewing PCOS not just as a biochemical disorder but as a mental issue I needed to overcome. Only when I began addressing my mental issues did the physical changes become in sync with how I viewed myself and the world. It was a tough process and there were not a lot of resources I can turn to which specifically cater to the mental health issues of women with PCOS.

This book was written out of all that pain and insecurity I have nurtured all through these years living with PCOS. Even just writing this book has become very therapeutic for me. This book is a product of all the experiences that have shaped how I approached and felt about PCOS. I emphasize that I am not a medical professional so I encourage you to check with your doctor first before trying out the things that I will be sharing with you. These learnings come from my own research, professional advices I received, interviews with other women and my own experiences. Rather than being restricted to this disorder, I offer readers, my fellow women with PCOS, a hope that we are more than this disorder. Whilst PCOS is largely a medical condition, I propose a more holistic approach to this disorder. Through this book, I am going to walk you through managing this condition medically, intellectually, physically, emotionally and perhaps even spiritually. As you start reading this, I welcome you to a journey that may be painful but ultimately rewarding. I think that there is already some form of healing done when we feel a sense of kinship and oneness even just by reading text about PCOS by women with PCOS.

Chapter 1

PCOS in a Nutshell

Even before we begin to define what PCOS is, perhaps it is good to assess our level of understanding at this point. How much do we really know about this disorder? How much are we willing to learn about it? You may have heard about PCOS because you may have been diagnosed with it. Or you may come across it because you have exhibited symptoms and a doctor, or a friend may have referred you to have yourself checked for this. In any case, the first real preparation you can do for encountering this disorder is on the level of the mind. You have to gauge how far you want to understand this disorder that will affect every aspect of you.

There are many levels of how people are willing to learn about PCOS. Some people are content with browsing articles online or recommended links from friends. They see something on a webpage that said 'PCOS' and they clicked it. Or a friend may have shared a good journal and you felt intrigued with the link. And some are already content with the information they get from this. The internet is really a treasure trove of information which is unparalleled. You may need not go to university just to learn things from the internet. But we should also be wary of the information we get from the internet. There are a lot of web resources passing off as the work of professionals and may convince ordinary readers about their credibility. To be fair, most of these websites have a general picture of what PCOS is. But you still have to sift through the information you get and see if this is authentic and scientific, or these are just marketing baits that will lead you to buy an assortment of drugs having therapeutic claims.

Others will go as far as trying to understand PCOS to the biochemical level. These people may be ordinary individuals who may not have a background in medicine, in research or even in basic sciences. I belong to this category, because I really didn't have a formal background in medicine. But the pain that I felt while experiencing PCOS drove me to become an expert about the disorder. I wanted to understand exactly how PCOS affects my body, down to the smallest unit. I guess, the level of understanding we may be open to depends on how far we have been affected by the disorder. If you feel that it is not bothersome, then internet articles may suffice for you. But if you are like me, suffering from the aches and pains of PCOS on an everyday basis, then you will want to extend your understanding a little bit deeper and more comprehensive than the normal person. I am not saying you should get a PhD on PCOS or enroll in a medical course. I am just saying that this book is a product of much research and personal experience that will touch on a lot of technical aspects of the disorder. In my experience, the more we know about something, the more we are able to have power over it. The less we have knowledge about something, the more power it has on us.

So, returning to our topic, polycystic ovarian syndrome or PCOS is medically defined as an endocrine disorder fulfilling at least two of the three Rotterdam criteria (2003)[2]:

- Oligomenorrhea or amenorrhea
- Signs of androgen excess
- Multiple ovarian cysts

Rotterdam criteria refer to the set of criteria made by scientific experts in 2003 to diagnose PCOS. The workshop was held in Rotterdam, Netherlands. This may be a mouthful of technical terms at this point. Some may not want to proceed after such terms are laid out. And I am warning you that things will still get technically complicated the more we discuss the medical part of this disorder. But I will do my best to explain the terms and references that ordinary people will understand. Again, I am a firm believer that understanding is key in healing, and that women with PCOS should do their best to understand their condition in order to seek the treatment they need. I promise you that I will discuss most of the scientific terms and processes in ways every one of us can understand. But you should not be averse to being challenged intellectually by such a disorder. Only with comprehensive understanding can there be any progress to healing.

Oligo- or amenorrhea are terms that refer to ovulation or that part of the month where you are most fertile. The term 'menorrhea' refers to menstruation, while the terms 'oligo' and 'a' refer to 'few' and 'no' respectively. Taken together, oligomenorrhea means few menstruation and amenorrhea means no menstruation. The activity of menstruation indicates that a woman is fertile or capable of reproduction. Hence, we can say that PCOS is largely a condition that affects women of reproductive age the most. When you have menses, you are considered to be in your reproductive years. We will discuss menstruation more thoroughly in the next parts. But at this point, it is sufficient to know that every month, a woman who has menstruated will be fertile or ovulating.

If a woman becomes pregnant, then the menses stop until the woman has given birth and after breastfeeding. If a woman does not become pregnant, menses commence as seen as the monthly bloody discharge. Oligo-ovulation then is a condition where you have fewer than 8 menstrual periods in a year. You should be having twelve menstrual periods in a year if you do not become pregnant. If you only have 8 menstrual periods during the year, then you might have PCOS or a disorder that prevents you from ovulating. Amenorrhea, on the other hand, refers to the condition where a woman does not have menses for three or more consecutive months. We emphasize here the modifier 'consecutive' because some women may miss a period for a month and then have their period on the next. In PCOS, the lack of menses should occur for three or more consecutive months.

It is important for you at this point to check your monthly menses. There are a lot of apps you can use so you can track your menstrual cycle. Women who are suspecting whether they have PCOS should be monitoring their periods closely. Sometimes, you may already have started menstruating, but you did not remember having one. Errors in logging menstruation may lead to under or over-diagnosis of PCOS.

The second criterion refers to signs of androgen excess. We will discuss more of these in the next chapter. But in brief, androgen is a hormone naturally produced by everyone, regardless of sex. But men tend to produce more androgen than women. This hormone is responsible for many of the manly features in males. Because of androgen and subsequently, testosterone, men tend to have more facial and body hair, have broader shoulders and lower voices. Women also express androgen but to a lesser degree than men. If there is an excess of androgen, women may have more hair on their face and body or even have lower voices than other women. We can see this in the appearance of women with PCOS or we can test the amount of androgen in their body to confirm the excess.

The last criterion is more of ultrasound diagnosis. You can only know if you have polycystic ovaries through ultrasound. And sometimes, this can be an accident, for example, you are having an ultrasound as a routine checkup or you are being checked for another disorder. Through some mechanism, hormones in your body contribute to the formation of these cysts surrounding your ovaries. You may not feel that you have polycystic ovaries because they don't present with specific symptoms. This criterion would only supplement the first two. You may not know that you have PCOS until you have yourself checked or you begin experiencing symptoms.

But the underlying definition of PCOS is that it is primarily an endocrinal disorder. The endocrine system may not be familiar to many readers who are not in the medical profession. You may have heard of other systems such as the skeletal, muscular, cardiovascular, respiratory, and digestive or nervous systems. The body is composed of these different systems which have a specific role in making sure that we are functioning well. For example, the cardiovascular system takes care of the heart and the blood vessels, making sure that we have an adequate supply of oxygen-rich blood in every part of our body. These systems are very much connected with each other. For example, the respiratory system takes care of delivering oxygen from the outside to the body, while the cardiovascular is responsible for distributing that oxygen to the body via our blood. The goal is that each system must be working in harmony with the other body systems.

The endocrine system has an important role in our body. It takes care of our hormones, or the internal communication system of our body. The endocrine system includes parts of your brain such as the hypothalamus and the pituitary, the adrenal glands on top of your kidneys, your pancreas and your sexual organs namely the testes and the ovaries. We will explain the function of the endocrine system in further detail in the next chapters. But suffice to say, the endocrine system affects all parts of your body. It is responsible for the release of your growth hormones which will induce your body to become bigger. The endocrine system regulates the amount of heat you have in your body when it releases your thyroid hormones. And in the case of PCOS, the endocrine system is responsible for regulating hormones necessary for sexual differentiation and reproduction.

So, when we say that the endocrine system involves all parts of the body, we are also saying that PCOS is a disorder that affects all parts of our bodies. Even if the only symptom you feel is that you don't have menses, the effect of PCOS will go beyond your sexual organs. We will discuss in another chapter how these different symptoms of PCOS come about because of the wide-reaching effect of the endocrine system. At this point, we just have to note how complex and comprehensive

PCOS can affect the body. It will affect your fertility and your capacity to have a baby. It will make a mark on your body size and your self-concept of that. It will affect your eating patterns and the choices of food you should be taking. It will change your skin and the way you come across other people. It will change your body and your health status from your pubertal years, to your reproductive years until your menopausal years. The endocrine system, though not as known as the others, underlies the potency of PCOS.

Hence, the treatment and management of PCOS must not only target specific symptoms of the disorder. There should also be a thorough study on how these existing medications affect other parts of the body which may not be the primary target of these drugs. Another chapter will deal more closely with treatment modalities. But we have to bear in mind that because PCOS is an endocrine disorder, we should be targeting a lot of organ systems at one time if we want to manage it. Only addressing one aspect of PCOS may contribute to the worsening of our symptoms. We also have to expand our understanding of health, not just as a physical condition, but also as a mental health issue. What we feel in our bodies become processes in our minds. And if the body is sick, the mind can also be sick. If we address only the body without heeding the mind, then we still remain sick. This book aims to make our understanding and management of PCOS as wide-reaching and comprehensive as the endocrine system.

Chapter 2

PCOS, Hormones and the Brain

You might be thinking that your ovaries involved in PCOS are down there in your pelvis. But I am saying that they are also affected by our brains up there. The connection may not be so apparent, but if we try to understand it, we could reach a profound appreciation of how our bodies can be so integrated and efficient. In this chapter, we are going to highlight how the brain and the hormones function to bring about PCOS and its symptoms. I apologize if this chapter might confuse you with so many technical terms or medical explanations. If you are averse to this or if you feel you are not ready to understand much of the medicine behind PCOS, you may opt to skip this part. But for those of you who really want to understand their condition and are willing to pay the price of hard labor and patience in order to fully appreciate the disorder, then soldier on. I will promise that I will ease the terms with you gently and with much explanation.

To start off, the human body is one of the most efficient systems in the world. This sophistication perhaps landed us on top of the food chain, as we are more efficient and sophisticated than other animals. Our bodies are capable of performing various functions. We have an intact repair mechanism when something malfunctions. We are able to think, adapt to situations, reproduce, protect ourselves from danger, and survive. And most importantly, we have an internal system of communication that enables the different parts of the body to communicate with each other. When there is a deficiency in one part, a signal is released so that other systems can address the problem. Together, the different parts of the body act as a whole in making us functional human beings.

One of the communication systems of the body is the endocrine system. The previous chapter gave us an overview of how this system affects

PCOS. In broad terms, the endocrine system makes sure that there is an adequate supply of needed hormones and nutrients in the body. We are able to assess the excess and deficiency in one part of our body through our endocrine system. Much of this communication happens without you being conscious of anything. That is why you might not feel your endocrine system too much until something goes wrong.

As we have mentioned in the previous chapter, the endocrine system involves specific parts of the body, the most important of which is the brain. The brain is made up of many parts that control various functions in our body. In terms of the endocrine system, the brain contains two centers governing the hormonal system: the hypothalamus and the pituitary gland. These two structures are way inside your brain so it may be hard to appreciate it, much less visualize it. The hypothalamus and the pituitary are like factories of signals. Within their structure, they manufacture the needed signals to be produced by the body. The direction of the signal is from the hypothalamus to the pituitary. The hypothalamus sends a message to the pituitary to produce a certain type of hormone. When the pituitary receives the message, it is going to produce the next set of messengers to target the organs who will produce the hormones themselves. For example, a growth releasing hormone is signaled from the hypothalamus. It will travel to your pituitary which will read the message and produce the next signal which is your growth hormones. These hormones will then travel through different parts of your body that will stimulate growth in your bones, your skin, your muscles and in major organs of the body.

We will only focus on the system directly involved in PCOS which is your reproductive system. Your body is able to regulate your reproductive hormones through your endocrine system. It will start with your hypothalamus which manufactures your gonadotropin-releasing hormones or GnRH. This may be a very technical term, but it only means a special kind of hormone that will induce your body to produce reproductive hormones. The pituitary will sense this signal and because of this, it will produce two kinds of hormones: your luteinizing hormones or LH and your follicle-stimulating hormones or FSH. Again, these may be two very technical terms, but they only mean two special kinds of reproductive hormones that have unique functions which I will explain in a few. The signal will then travel through the body via our blood. When it reaches your ovaries, the signal will now be finally read and executed.

Now, the ovary is the main reproductive organ of the woman. It contains all the eggs needed by the woman to conceive a child. It will release an egg from one of the two ovaries once a month. The ovary is a special kind of organ because it will also produce the hormones needed for reproduction. When the luteinizing hormone or LH reaches the ovary, it will stimulate special areas in the ovary, specifically your theca cells. Once the theca cells are activated, it will transform the cholesterol floating in your blood into androstenedione or your androgen. This androgen is responsible for giving women certain masculine features like the hair in their pubic area or even acne. We also see how cholesterol plays an important part in the hormone systems. Actually, reproductive hormones all come from cholesterol. The body simply modifies the cholesterol to form different kinds of hormones. In the case of your theca cells, they will convert cholesterol into androgen, the masculinizing hormone.

You might think, wait, why does the woman produce masculinizing hormones if they are women? Well, this is simply a natural occurrence that everyone, men and women alike, produce both masculinizing and feminizing hormones. The difference is only in the production of the major hormones. Men produce androgen and testosterone in greater proportion than estrogen that is why they have more masculine features. Women produce more estrogen than testosterone that is why they have more feminizing features. But the fact that both sexes produce both hormones reflects how many similarities we share with each other. Some men have higher voices than others and this might be because they produce more estrogen than other men. Some women have more hair in their face because they produce more androgen or testosterone. The difference only lies in the more dominantly produced hormone.

On the other hand, when the follicle-stimulating hormone reaches the ovaries through your granulosa cells, it will convert the androgen that your theca cell produces into estrogen. Here, we already see the link between the two hormones. One type of cell, the theca cell, will produce the androgen. The granulosa cells, on the other hand, will use that androgen and convert it to estrogen. The granulosa cells need androgen first before they can make estrogen, like some sort of a base substance that they can transform. If you are not able to produce androgens, then the granulosa cells cannot produce the estrogen. This estrogen is the main reproductive hormone for women. Estrogen is responsible for endowing you with female features.

As compared to men, women have curvier lips, higher pitch voices, and delicate features. Estrogen is also responsible for making you fertile and able to reproduce. Some effects of estrogen also include endowing your body with protection from heart problems and it can also strengthen your bones.

The estrogen you produce is very much dependent on the number of eggs in your ovaries. Since you have a fixed number of eggs produced over a lifetime, your production of estrogen will also be very limited. You will begin having more feminine features when you menstruate. This coincides with the release of the first eggs from your ovaries in puberty. Once you begin menstruating, your ovaries will now regularly release one egg from your ovaries once a month. When they are fertilized, then pregnancy will ensue. But when they are not, the unfertilized egg will create a signal that will make you menstruate. The cycle repeats again as your uterus prepares for another monthly round of expectant fertilization.

Once you have reached the limit of the number of eggs released, you will undergo a phase called menopause, literally halting your menstruation into a pause. Without the eggs in your ovaries, you will not be able to produce much estrogen. Without estrogen, the body will feel the classic symptoms of menopause, including heat flushes, brittle bones, and dryness in your genital organs. All of these happen as a consequence of the natural course of your reproductive system.

Now, we can see how the brain and the reproductive organs work. A signal from your hypothalamus will reach your pituitary. The pituitary will release two kinds of hormones, the luteinizing and the follicle-stimulating hormones. These two will reach your ovaries and form your androgen which will be converted to your estrogen. Your brain initiates a cascade of messages that results in the production of your reproductive hormones.

But it does not stop there. The hypothalamus-pituitary-ovarian system is not a one-way street but actually a loop. The ovaries have a way of sending a message back to the brain. When there is an excess of androgen or estrogen in your system, the message will travel through your blood and reach your brain. The hypothalamus in the brain will sense the increased levels of these hormones and will conclude that there are enough hormones needed by the body. It will then stop producing the first signal, halting the cascade of events. The hormones then in your body is controlled through this process called the 'negative feedback.' The body can sense if there are enough hormones in your system so that you don't produce more than you need. We can say that our bodies are really efficient because it has this capacity to regulate its own without producing waste products. From the hypothalamus to the pituitary to the ovaries, a signal will once again go to your hypothalamus thus restarting the cycle again.

How does PCOS work in this endocrine system? PCOS is primarily seen as a failure in the feedback mechanism of your hypothalamus-pituitary-ovarian system. In PCOS, there is a problem with the signal from your hypothalamus to your pituitary. Certain factors such as genetics, stress, diet, radiation exposure or other environmental stressors can change the amount and rhythm of signals from your hypothalamus to your pituitary. When this occurs, the pituitary will also send out an abnormal signal. Instead of releasing both luteinizing and follicle-stimulating hormones, there is now a preference for the production of more luteinizing hormones only. This will cascade all the way to your ovaries. If you only have luteinizing hormones, then you will only produce androgen. This will now be reflected in the first criterion of PCOS as your androgen excess. We will see in the next chapter how these manifests in your body as the symptoms of PCOS. But basically, you will have more masculinizing features because of the androgen excess. The ovaries will try to send a signal to your hypothalamus regarding this excess. Completing the abnormal cycle, the ovaries will send a signal regarding the excess of your androgen and the lack of your estrogen. The hypothalamus will interpret this as a need to produce more hormones and will release more messengers to produce an abnormal number of hormones. The vicious cycle of PCOS is then perpetuated.

We mentioned in the previous paragraph how certain factors affect the abnormal cascade of hormones in the hypothalamus-pituitary-ovarian system. The actual cause of PCOS is unknown. There are studies which explore the higher incidence of PCOS among siblings and family members who have PCOS. If you have a mother or a sister that have PCOS, you have a higher chance of getting PCOS than the normal population. Men are also not spared from the genetic effects of PCOS. Men with relatives who have PCOS have been found out to have early balding and insulin resistance compared to the general male population. Further studies in the exact genomic variations on PCOS are currently underway.

This chapter may have been a mouthful for you. There are so many technical terms and processes mentioned about PCOS and the endocrine system. When I first tried learning about PCOS in the medical sense, I was also very confused about the different hormones and the signaling system. I even felt discouraged from learning because of the complexity of the systems involved. But the more that I pushed myself in learning about PCOS, the more PCOS made sense. I began to have a profound respect for doctors and how they are able to explain my symptoms of PCOS. And with knowledge comes greater confidence in dealing with this disorder. The hardest part in the learning process is over, but there are still more to come in the next chapters.

Chapter 3

Symptoms of PCOS

How do we know that a woman has PCOS? There are a significant number of women who may manifest some symptoms of PCOS but disregard them as though what they are feeling is just normal. The lack of understanding of how PCOS manifests leads to the danger of delayed diagnosis. When we don't know what PCOS is and how it is seen in women, we may not seek the necessary help we may need. These symptoms are universal but will vary per person. The degree of one symptom may be more intense in another compared to others. Nevertheless, we still follow the Rotterdam criteria of amenorrhea, androgen excess and polycystic ovaries in diagnosing PCOS. Here are just some symptoms of PCOS we should be able to identify easily. I will try to relate each symptom to the medical learnings we gained from the previous chapters.

Irregular Periods and Infertility

As we have mentioned, the primary criterion of PCOS is seen in the irregular menstruation of women. Follicle-stimulating hormone is needed to induce the ovaries to release an egg each month. In PCOS, there is less or even zero production of the follicle-stimulating hormone. Thus, the release of eggs or ovulation may be unpredictable. In one month, the woman could ovulate through a minimal adequate amount of follicle-stimulating hormone. In another month, no ovulation may occur. The ovulation of a woman then signifies her fertility. The more consistent the ovulation per month is, the higher the chances the woman can get pregnant if unprotected sexual intercourse happens.

In PCOS then, the fertility of a woman is compromised. PCOS women have a harder time getting pregnant because the lack of adequate amounts of follicle-stimulating hormone does not ripe their ovaries to release an egg. It is still possible to get pregnant if some follicle-stimulating hormone is produced, however small an amount. But the odds are not against women with PCOS. This can be very frustrating for women who want to get pregnant. I want to reiterate that having PCOS does not mean you are infertile. I am only emphasizing that it is harder for women with PCOS to get pregnant.

Without ovulation, menstruation is also compromised. When a woman ovulates, the released egg sends signals to the uterus to prepare for making the egg viable for pregnancy. The uterus does this by thickening its membranes. At the peak of ovulation, the uterus is thick enough to supply the egg with enough nutrients. When a sperm is able to fertilize the egg, then the uterus undergoes a series of changes that will prepare the body for pregnancy. But if there is no sperm to fertilize the egg, the signal from the egg to the uterus is halted. The thickened membrane of the uterus is shed off and seen as your monthly blood discharge. When you don't have ovulation as in the case of PCOS, there is no signal for the uterus to thicken and be shed off. So, there may be months when you don't have your bloody discharge.

There are reports of women with PCOS who complain of heavy and irregular bleeding at times. This occurs more often in women who have heavier weights. The excess androgen they produce from the predominance of the luteinizing hormone is converted by your cholesterol or fats in other parts of the body including your hips, your stomach, your arms, and legs, into some form of estrogen. If there is more androgen and if there is more cholesterol in a woman, then there is more estrogen circulating in the body. With increased estrogen, the uterus may thicken. The thickening of the uterus is not due to the released egg in ovulation, but by the peripheral conversion of your androgen to your estrogen. The thickened uterus may be shed off irregularly and this is seen as the abnormal heavy bleeding some women with PCOS experience. You should go to your OB-Gyn when you feel heavy and unpredictable vaginal bleeding at any point.

But not all women who have irregular periods have PCOS. In fact, around 50% of women who have started menstruating will have some episodes of irregular periods[3]. This is because their hypothalamus-pituitary-ovarian system is just developing. You may then diagnose a teenager with irregular periods as a case of PCOS. But it is more prudent to wait a while until after 18 years of age. At this point, the body should have developed its reproductive system to its full maturity. If there are irregular periods still, then we can begin entertaining the possibility of PCOS.

Excessive Hair

We have repeatedly stated that in PCOS, the luteinizing hormone produces excess androgen in a woman's body. Androgen is responsible for the masculine features in people. If there is an excess of androgen, then the person is endowed with more masculine features.

When the androgen hormones encounter hair follicles, this will stimulate the growth of coarse and dark terminal hairs. The hair thickening follows a particular pattern seen in men. These areas are called your androgen-sensitive areas. When androgen reaches these sites, then the coarse dark hair will be more developed in these areas. The excessive hair growth can then be seen in the upper lip, chin, sideburns, chest and the area below the umbilicus. You might see some women with a faint mustache on their lips or a furry growth in the chest. You may then suspect that they have androgen excess and you may entertain the idea of PCOS.

The pubic area is also the site of excessive hair growth. Though they both have hair, the pattern of hair distribution is different in men and women. Men will have a more diamond-shaped pubic hair distribution, from the belly button to the pelvic areas. In women, the pattern is more triangle-shaped, starting from the base in the mons pubis to the vaginal area. In PCOS, the hair pattern in women becomes more of a diamond shape.

Having unwanted hair in your body may be a cause of shame for some women. They may seek ways on how to reduce body hair, from drinking medication or shaving the hair completely. The anxiety is but natural since we all want to look presentable and attractive. But the excess hair could affect our body-image making us more self-conscious and insecure. This could be a starting point of some psychological issues regarding body image in PCOS.

In women of more advanced age, the thinning of hair can be a major issue. Alopecia is the technical term used to describe hair loss seen as thinning of hair with preservation of the hairline. Again, this is due to androgen excess in women with PCOS. The thinning of hair can often be embarrassing as the pattern may start from the top of the head. The gaps in hair patches may be more obvious through time and women may resort to either wearing wigs or shaving it completely. But it may not happen to all women with PCOS.

Acne and Other Skin Issues

One of the most pertinent issues in women, especially of the adolescent age, is the proliferation of acne. All adolescents undergo this ugly phase of acne formation. It is one of the most visible signs that a child is transitioning to adolescents. Teenagers often seek ways, however drastic, to reduce their acne. From facial rubs to skin cleansers to pimple patches, teenagers are the favorite target of cosmetic companies. And the disappearance of acne may mark a shift to adulthood. But in some cases, the acne in women with PCOS can be persistent even thru their adult years.

Again, we will blame androgen excess for the persistence of acne in women with PCOS. The skin contains a particular type of gland called your sebaceous glands. This is responsible mainly for keeping your skin pores tight and warm as they produce your sebum or your oil. When you notice that your face is quite oily, your sebaceous glands are actively secreting your sebum. In androgen excess, the androgen hormones stimulate your sebaceous glands to produce more sebum. You will feel oilier in the process. When there is excess sebum, the oil can make the area prone to infiltration of bacteria called the *Propionibacterium acnes,* found in your skin. The skin will be irritated with this bacteria proliferation and will mount a defense to combat it. This results in inflammation, seen as reddening and thickening of the skin. Taken together, there is excess oil, with the proliferation of your bacteria and inflammation, seen then as your acne outbreak. In PCOS, because there is an androgen excess, there is the persistence of the acne even thru adulthood.

Like the issue with excess hair, acne can affect self-image dramatically. Overuse of skin products may often result in aggravating the problem instead of solving it. Some of these symptoms can actually just be solved by proper handwashing and liberate washing of your face with plain soap and water. But as the acne persists, the insecurity of women with PCOS increases.

One strange skin condition some women with PCOS experience is called *acanthosis nigricans*. This is seen as thickened, grey-brown velvety skin tags in your neck, armpits, waist, and groin area and underneath the breasts. *Acanthosis nigricans* is more common in women with PCOS who are obese compared to others. It may be a sore sight for some as though you are infected with some disorder. You might try to cover up for the unsightly skin tags and brown creases through a number of products.

Acanthosis nigricans can be more related to the other prevalent endocrine disorder in PCOS called insulin resistance. We will discuss it more in another chapter. But in brief, the skin discoloration is a product of excess in your insulin. This is seen more in diabetic patients but *acanthosis nigricans* is not exclusively a reflection of PCOS or diabetes. It may also signify other diseases involving your digestive system. When you notice these skin discolorations, it might be good to consult a doctor for a work-up.

Weight Gain

A lot of women with PCOS complain of weight gain. They are significantly heavier than most women, but not all heavy-sized women have PCOS. The term 'weight gain' might also be too general for us to use in our discussion of PCOS. Would a weight gain of 1kg already make one think of PCOS? We will use a classification system for weight that is used in medicine and may be more politically correct at this point. We can begin discussing weight more in terms of body mass index or BMI. Your BMI would reflect the proportion of your height with your weight. You can compute for your BMI using the following formula:

$$BMI = Weight\ (in\ kilograms)\ /\ Height\ (in\ meters)^2$$

According to the World Health Organization[4], the BMI of a person will signify a person's certain state of health. If you have a BMI below 18.5 kg/m², then you are considered underweight. A normal BMI will fall between a BMI of 18.5 – 24.9 kg/m². A BMI of 25-29.9kg/m² is considered overweight, a score of 30-34.9 kg/m² means obese Type 1 and a score of 35 to 39.9 kg/m² is obese Type II. A BMI score of more than 40 kg/m² is termed 'morbidly obese'. A good proportion of women with PCOS fall into the overweight to obese categories.

We will have a more thorough discussion of how weight gain works in the chapter on insulin resistance. But in brief, women with PCOS have a tendency to point on more weight compared to other women. It is not because they eat too much, although that may be the case for some. But more than the amount of food we eat, the problem lies in how the body stores the food that we eat. Women with PCOS have a harder time shedding off their weight because the food is stored in their bodies as fat. They are more prone to store that body fat which deposits mainly in the waist and in the arms and legs. Even with exercise, the body still has a difficult time burning all that stored fat.

We have to emphasize here that it is not because women with PCOS eat bad fatty food that is why they are heavy-sized. There are a lot of people without PCOS who are overweight and obese. The problem with PCOS is not just in the amount of food they eat, but what our body does to the food. Instead of using the food as an energy source and excreting away the excess, women with PCOS will store the food in a more prolonged manner. Therefore, there is extra effort to control what we eat as well as maintain an active lifestyle that will burn those fats away.

Obstructive Sleep Apnea

What happens when we snore? When we sleep, most of the muscles in our body are limp and relax. This is to allow our muscles to rest. Our throat and the back of our mouth are also muscles that rest when we sleep. As they are resting, they may tend to block the air flow from our mouth to our throat to the lungs. This obstruction to the airflow is heard as a sound, that of snoring.

Women with PCOS are prone to snoring. As they sleep, the muscles in their throat and the back of their mouth tend to relax, obstructing the airflow and producing the characteristic sound of snoring. But since they also have a lot of stored fat, there is greater obstruction in the throat area, increasing the tension of airflow. This is called your obstructive sleep apnea. If you have heard somebody really snoring very loudly, then you may suspect obstructive sleep apnea. Because there is not enough air going in through our body when there is that obstruction, the tendency of the body is really to breathe harder and faster. Though this is not a medical emergency, you should still see a doctor. The fat deposits may reach a point of totally occluding your airway and you may have difficulty breathing even during waking hours.

Mood, Depression, and Anxiety

The issue of mental health in PCOS is not something that is thoroughly discussed in medical books or scientific journals. People take for granted that PCOS is just an endocrine disorder involving the reproductive system or your body size. But all of these changes affect your mental health, contributing further to the physical disorder. In fact, mental health issues are more difficult to treat because they are often underreported. But all these changes brought about by your endocrine system warrant a thorough look at your mental health.

Women with PCOS have a higher tendency for some psychiatric disorders. A lot of these results from the undesirable body image. Having a lot of unwanted hair, sprouting pimples, having difficulty getting pregnant and being obese all contribute to a negative self-image. There is a tendency to compare yourself with other women and from social standards of beauty. These self-images may then affect even your mood and general outlook. Some may even feel depressed about how they look. A lot will feel anxious about appearing in public or dating potential life partners. We will discuss all these psychiatric disorders more thoroughly in another chapter. But we can say that physical changes brought about by PCOS will affect our mental health.

We also said in the chapter on PCOS and the brain that stress plays a role in the imbalance in signaling. When there is too much stress that you experience, certain stress hormones are produced which interfere with the natural signal of the hypothalamus to the pituitary to the ovaries and back. The vicious cycle of PCOS is perpetuated by the unnecessary stress we lead our bodies to experience. Stress can come from the negative self-image we have and the social pressure we feel. The more we detest our bodies and how we look like, the more stressed we become. The more we feel anxious to fit in the standards of society in terms of beauty and health, the more stressed we become. The higher the stress level, the higher the risk of negatively affecting the endocrine system. Thus,

PCOS is reinforced by the stress that caused it. When we begin to see that the vicious cycle need not continue, then hope for curing PCOS is possible.

Long Term Effects

Most of these changes happen across the adolescent stage to adulthood. During the first few years, there may be active attempts to address the specific issues of PCOS like hair excess, obesity or acne. You may find yourselves buying and putting on tons of products on your body just to cure each symptom of PCOS. But after a while, the symptoms still persist despite the medications you try out. There is a sense of hopelessness that you feel, hence you stop trying to find a solution out of the problems PCOS inflicts on you. With ignorance, the petty problems you may have can actually have long term effects that have the potential to physically and emotionally harm you.

Consider obesity, when you stop trying to lose weight because your previous efforts have not paved off, then you will keep on putting on weight.

With increased weight, a lot of cardiovascular diseases can develop. The increased cholesterol you eat and not burn off will deposit in various parts of your body including your blood vessels. Through time, these cholesterol deposits will accumulate and even partially block your vessels. This is felt as hypertension, when your body exceeds extra effort to circulate blood through occluded blood vessels. When the cholesterol deposit totally blocks the vessels, you are at a greater risk of a heart attack or even a stroke, depending on where the block happens. These cardiovascular events do not happen within a week or a month. The fats deposit through a lot of years of neglect. You may think that dieting and exercising is a losing game. But if you continue binging and being careless at what kind of foods you eat, then you are increasing your chances of developing harmful diseases earlier.

If you do not address your mental health issues, then you also run the risk of a mental health breakdown. When you ignore symptoms like depression or anxiety, thinking that it is just normal and that you can get over it on your own, then you may fall deeper into your own issues. You may run the risk of suicidal ideation when you feel that the pressure to look better gets the better of you. You may have panic attacks that prevent you from living the life that you want. These will also affect your physical health. When you feel too much stress, you may also run the risk of developing cardiovascular diseases. Stresses creates a lot of reactive oxygen species, substances that destroy your system from within. When the mind suffers, the body will suffer more.

In terms of the lack of menstruation, you may feel more pressured that you won't become pregnant. The more you feel anxious about not ovulating, the more you will not get pregnant. There may be two schools of thought in this respect. On the one hand, negative thinking is self-fulfilling. The more that you think that you will not be able to do something, the more that it will not happen. Self-fulfilling prophecies already doom you even before you try doing something about it. On the other hand, a biochemical approach to infertility can also be explained by stress. When you feel too much stress as you think about getting pregnant, the more haywire the signaling system in your hypothalamus-pituitary-ovarian axis will be. Stress hormones will interfere with the normal signaling and thus, you will really develop infertility. From a simple lack of menstruation, you may now face a lot of challenges in terms of your relationship with your partner as well as your dreams of forming your own biological family.

It is important for us to see how symptoms of PCOS play out as a spectrum, increasing in intensity and complexity through the years. You might only be dealing with acne in your adolescence. But later on, this may develop into negative self-concepts that will perpetuate your depression. If you do not address the small issues when they start, then they will simply morph into undefeatable monsters later on. You have to accept that PCOS is not something you cure overnight or even in a few years. You need to change your perspective about PCOS in a radical way by thinking of long-term solutions instead of Band-Aid remedies. Nobody gets cured of PCOS in a year. But you can prevent PCOS from totally ruining your life when you begin to accept that you must change in terms of how you think and feel about your disorder. I still have PCOS even though I have been diagnosed with it a long time ago. But I have learned to steer clear of the detrimental effects of PCOS in the long term because I addressed the small issues earlier on. Detecting PCOS at an earlier stage will help you prepare yourself in combating its long-term effects. With an earlier diagnosis, you can actually seek help earlier on.

Chapter 4

PCOS as a Woman Ages

PCOS is a condition that you grow with. Unlike diseases like pneumonia or hepatitis, PCOS is not a one-time, temporary disorder that you can purge away with medications. It is a disorder that will affect you from your teenage years and well into your menopausal years. It is important to understand this early on because you may be very frustrated at trying out several medications and still failing to address the symptoms of PCOS. If you begin to see PCOS as a multi-headed monster that you can only manage, but never totally cure, then you can begin setting more realistic expectations. In this chapter, I have tried to chronicle some of my experiences growing up with PCOS. Though these experiences may vary amongst women, the general trend of hormone excess and diminishment will more or less be the same. I will still incorporate medical terms to aid us in understanding these changes further. By seeing PCOS as a lifelong condition, we may begin to show some respect to the formidable enemy we have to live with.

Young children may not experience the symptoms of PCOS yet. We have repeatedly emphasized how PCOS is an abnormality in the endocrine system, specifically in the hypothalamus-pituitary-ovarian loop. In young children, this axis is not yet fully developed because of immature organs that are not yet capable of exerting a visible effect on the body. Thus, it is not wise to start screening kids for PCOS. Young girls may look chubby, but it is not a predictor of having PCOS.

The moment a young girl reaches her menses, the beginning signs of PCOS can be observed. With a maturing endocrine system, the hormones are now exerting visible changes in a girl's body. Because of the production of estrogen, girls will start seeing their breasts budding with their nipples forming a distinct mound. Pubic hair is also starting to crop up, assuming the familiar triangular shape in the pelvis. Pubertal changes can be very dramatic at this point. The limit is reached when the young girl has her first menses. This marks the start of the monthly release of the egg. The average age this happens is around 12 to 13 years of age and girls may expect their monthly period to occur, if no sexual contact has been successful to fertilize their egg[5]. There may be times that the menses are not regular. And this is still normal because the endocrine system is not fully mature. There will be times when you miss your menses for a month, and then regain it again on the third. There could even be large gaps in months between menses. While this may be alarming and may warrant a consult, the diagnosis of PCOS should not be hastily made. We say that after 18 years of age, the endocrine system of young women are quite mature enough. Any irregular periods after that age of maturity may indicate PCOS or other disorders. There is just increased index of suspicion because PCOS is one of the most common conditions for the lack of menstruation.

In the adolescent age, the physical changes are accompanied by a lot of social and mental adjustments. The changes in height, shape, breast size and hair may be stressful for many teenagers. The eruption of acne also accompanies this stage of puberty. Girls will tend to compare themselves with each other. They are undergoing different stages of growth and development but the social pressure to be more beautiful and pleasing can be heightened. Not everyone will proceed in the same phase. Others may go through puberty at an earlier stage and some at a more advanced age. Genetics may be more to blame for this variation. But mentally, this can affect girls and how they see themselves. Issues like social anxiety and depression can already start taking root at this point. The standards set by social media and peer groups can be very pressuring for any teenager.

Social relationships are also a significant life event for teenagers. The range of intimacy can swing from classmates and acquaintances to best friends, girl gangs and sororities to exclusive relationships. Dating will start at this awkward stage as people try to test the limits of their social skills. The issue of gender will also start to be problematized at this point. Girls will question whether they want boys or other women. The gender orientation is in the process of becoming identified at this stage.

Now, women with PCOS will have to navigate through all these concerns. They may not be diagnosed yet with PCOS, but they will certainly feel some of the physical symptoms early on. They will develop emotional and mental mechanisms to cope with the physical changes. It is important for teenage girls to adopt healthy ways of coping with such changes. They must be able to have the inner strength to navigate the different changes as well as external support from friends who will reassure them through the awkwardness. If they are not able to develop mature adaptations, these issues will persist and affect them later on in life.

During adulthood, women with PCOS will have prominent symptoms of menstrual and ovarian dysfunction. It is assumed that after 18 years of age, the body has enough time to develop all its organs. Thus, irregular menses may already signify some endocrinal problems, and a primary consideration is PCOS. As women begin to enter into relationships with men, the formation of families becomes the concern in adulthood. Fertility then will be a primary challenge for women with PCOS. Again, we emphasize that having PCOS will not automatically mean that you are infertile. There is still some amount of follicle-stimulating hormone produced, though in small amounts. But that also means fertility is possible though the chance is slim.

In their first year of marriage, couples will try to have a baby and a first consult at a fertility clinic is anticipated. Couples will try to seek professional help in terms of conceiving a child. Doctors then may prescribe various medications including oral combined progesterone that are meant to induce menstruation and ovulation. Though this may be effective in some women, there should be a general note on the side effects of these medications. They are effective in bringing about menstruation, but you also have to watch out for adverse effects such as nausea, headaches, breast pain, weight gain, and mood changes.

When all pregnancy attempts have failed, couples will have to face a decision whether to stay in the marriage or break-up, live together childless or explore the possibility of adoption. All these frustrations can be very stressful to both husbands and wives. The effect of PCOS is not just a woman's problem, but a couple's dilemma. Men should be educated about PCOS lest they start blaming the woman for not being fertile. We have to make our partners aware that it is not our choice not to have children, but it is a biological impairment we need to overcome. The values of the couple are also tested at this point. Will they stay even if they don't have babies? Or is having a baby the deal breaker? The decision making will be very complex at this point that is why PCOS should not be viewed just as a medical condition. It will affect every part of your relationship with yourself and others.

Career is also an issue during adulthood. We cannot deny that physical appearance plays a big role in the work that we do. Even if we are content about how our body looks, some people will be very judgmental and apply standards that may seem unreasonable. Women with PCOS will have to struggle through these challenges in the work and social life.

With insulin resistance, women with PCOS will have difficulty losing weight. Unwanted hair may be very obvious and acne can be uncontrolled. All these physical factors may affect the work and social life of women. While companies will ideally try to go past these physical characteristics, the reality is that they don't. Women with PCOS have to struggle extra hard to prove themselves compared to their skinnier or smoother counterparts. Intelligence, patience and hard work are level playing fields and women with PCOS should exploit that. In time, there is a sense of acceptance and even confidence in how we look at ourselves. Our physical characteristics should not define us. We should start seeing how truly beautiful we are and not just how people would like to define us.

Menopause determines another landmark in a woman. Medically speaking, menopause is the cessation of menstruation for twelve consecutive months[6]. This happens around the age of 50 for most women around the world. Again, some women will have menopause earlier or later than this age. But it will come to everyone at some point. In menopause, the ovaries have exhausted all their eggs and are not capable of releasing any more. Without an egg, there are no hormones produced that will thicken the endometrium and be shed off as menstruation. Estrogen will be markedly decreased at this point. Symptoms of menopause include hot flashes as the temperature center of the woman's body adjusts to the lack of estrogen. Bones are also becoming more brittle as estrogen has previously played a major role in strengthening it.

In the case of PCOS, there has already been the lack of ovulation at the very beginning. So, symptoms of lack of menstruation are not getting any worse and may even improve as you age. Unlike women without PCOS, we have a tendency to still have estrogen even without the release of an egg. Remember that the excess androgen we have is converted peripherally into estrogen from our fat cells. This estrogen may keep the endometrium thick, but it will also mean having breakthrough bleeding. You should really see an OB-Gyn once you start noticing any sort of bleeding during your menopausal years. We want to watch out for any malignant growth in the pelvic area.

Long term effects of PCOS are also prominent in the menopausal years. The insulin resistance brings about gaining excess fat in your body. With an increase in fat, you will now feel the impact of hypertension. A medical consult is needed to start you on anti-hypertensive medication which may already be lifetime if uncontrolled. You will have to watch out for complications of hypertension including a heart attack or a stroke. If you have not been very careful as you age, your body will feel all sorts of pain all over.

Diabetes is also a big issue in menopause. We will discuss this more thoroughly in the chapter on insulin resistance. But having diabetes will complicate your other cardiovascular conditions. Complications of uncontrolled diabetes may lead you to worry about your eyes, your kidney, and your nerves. Cataracts in the eyes, diabetic nephropathy in the kidneys and diabetic neuropathy in the nerves may develop if you don't regulate your sugar. Having PCOS does not doom you to automatically have diabetes, but it simply raises the risk of you developing diabetes.

If you are able to control hypertension and diabetes threat in your menopausal years, they say that PCOS actually gets better as you age. The different changes in your hormonal output become level with those women without PCOS, making the playing field level. There are still the usual signs of menopause such as mood swings, hot flushes, brittle bones, and general frailty. There might even be less of the androgen excess in time. Though these physical changes are very much welcome, I found that it is the personal maturity one gains that make menopausal women with PCOS more at ease with our condition. The long years that I battled PCOS has made me less anxious about an instant cure or a temporary fix. Instead of crash diets or bombarding myself with medication, I have learned that maintaining a healthy lifestyle is a better approach to PCOS. Believe me, I tried all those skincare products to cure my hair excess and acne. I signed up for various fitness programs thinking I would slim fast. These methods work, but only for some time. The symptoms would recur after two weeks of not using these products. And the return would be even more depressing since my expectations for myself have been set on high standards. The cycle of hopelessness mimics the vicious endocrine cycle in PCOS. When I began accepting PCOS as a lifelong condition, I began to be gentler on myself. I realized that I don't need to depend on artificial products or suicidal diet and exercise regiments. I discovered a formula on approaching PCOS that I want to share with you and I have catered it for people with PCOS.

Chapter 5

Insulin Resistance and Diabetes

I will be devoting two chapters on food and nutrition just to emphasize the importance of this aspect in PCOS. The subject of food is central to any understanding of PCOS. We know from the previous chapters that PCOS is primarily an endocrinal abnormality governing the hypothalamus-pituitary-ovarian loop. But the effect of PCOS reaches far more than just this axis. There are studies that also correlate PCOS with insulin resistance which may eventually lead to diabetes. I am warning you that this chapter would get technical once again as we encounter a lot of medical terms. But if you have been through the previous chapters, you will be able to pick up faster because the hormones acting on the digestion and absorption of food relatively work in the same way as the other hormones we've discussed.

First, let me introduce you the main characters in this endocrinal system. There will be two important hormones governing food and nutrition in our body: insulin and glucagon. These are both produced in your pancreas, an organ in your abdominal area located at the back. These two hormones will have an effect on your whole body especially your liver, the muscles and your fats. They will tell your body if you are in a 'fed' state, which means that you are nourished and supplied with adequate nutrients or in a 'fasting' state, which means that you are undernourished and would need to eat more.

We can understand how these hormones work by tracing the path of food in our bodies. The journey starts with the food that we eat. More than giving us a good feeling, the true purpose of food is to provide the body with enough energy to do its functions. The composition of our food basically falls into three categories: fat, proteins and carbohydrates. All of these provide energy to our body and this is computed in calories. We will go through the nitty-gritty of calculating caloric requirements in the next chapter. But at this point, it is important for us to note that we have a minimum number of calories needed for maintaining daily function and that all foods provide different amounts of calories. We will go through each food group one at a time.

First, carbohydrates are the major component in our diet. In terms of the three food groups, carbohydrates are the fastest sources of energy. This means that if you need to exercise or respond to a threat, your body will use your carbohydrates stores faster than your proteins and fats. Carbohydrates fall into two categories: simple and complex. These terms usually just refer to the biochemical composition of the food. Simple carbohydrates are molecularly composed of simple sugars arranged in a uniform manner. Complex carbohydrates are molecularly composed of many kinds of simple sugars arranged in a variety of complex ways. It may be difficult to visualize it, but a simple explanation would be that when you view a simple carbohydrate in a microscope, it may look like a straight line. If you look at a complex carbohydrate in a microscope, you may see the semblance of an octopus.

Your simple carbohydrates or sugars, when broken down, are composed of simple molecules connected to each other. As such, they are easier to digest and absorb. They provide the fastest source of energy for the body. Simple sugars come from your fruits, dairy products, honey, and syrup. They are usually blended into your desserts giving you the 'sugar rush.'

Complex carbohydrates or sugars are composed of many simple sugar molecules which are attached in complex ways. As such, the body will need more time to break them down into useable resources. Complex carbohydrates include your starches such as bread, rice and pasta, grains like corn and rye, root vegetables like potatoes and beans.

Another classification of your sugars is whether they are refined or unrefined. Refinement refers to the process of processing your food so that you take away a lot of vitamins, minerals, and fibers from the food to make the calories more concentrated. As the names suggest, refined sugars are highly processed food like your candies and sweeteners and cakes. They are usually canned or undergo treatment in a factory to preserve their longevity. You can easily spot them on grocery shelves with a lot of preservatives and added chemical contents. They will provide your body with the same amount of calories as the other foods. But they will give you less of the vitamins, minerals, and fibers you need. Unrefined sugars or carbohydrates refer to unprocessed foods, those that grow organically and sold in markets. They contain the necessary vitamins, minerals and fiber you need, but may be digested slower than the refined sugars. It may be simplistic to say that refined sugars are your 'bad sugars' while the unprocessed ones are the 'good sugars'. But this may be a shortcut to understanding how we should be eating more natural foods rather than factory-made, highly refined products. The refining process strips food away from their additive nutrients while increasing the sugar in your blood. Our modern diet is composed more of these refined carbohydrates because they taste better than unprocessed food. But in the long run, these may be more toxic when taken in excess.

The second food group are fats. These are composed of complex molecules made from fatty acids and glycerol. Like carbohydrates, they also provide energy for the body. But unlike carbohydrates, fats are digested slower, absorbed slower and are used up by the body as energy at a later time. Think of fats are your reserved energy stores, like a generator kicking in only when the original supply of energy runs out. So, during exercise, your body is going to use up your carbohydrates first. When that supply runs out, your body is going to burn your fats so that you still get the energy you need. So, when the fat is not being used up, it will be stored in your body, accumulate and deposit in certain areas such as your hips, belly, breast, thighs and arms. A positive way of looking at large-sized bodies is to view them having a vast amount of unused energy. When viewed this way, you will be more motivated to use these resources into productive use.

They are also more efficient than the other food groups in terms of energy source. For each gram of fat that you eat, you will gain 9 calories. Proteins and carbohydrates, on the other hand, will give you only 4 calories per gram. That means, you will need to burn less fat to provide you with the same amount of energy provided by more carbohydrates and proteins.

Certain kinds of fats are needed to provide nutrition for a number of bodily processes. They provide fatty acids which are used to build up cells and nourish your brain. Fats also contain the base materials with which to form your hormones. Foods rich with Omega 3-fatty acids will reduce the risk for atherosclerosis or the clogging of your blood vessels with fat that might lead to a heart attack or a stroke. Examples of these include your fish and sunflower oil.

Like carbohydrates, fats can also be classified by the composition of their molecules. Saturated fats are kinds of fat that are solid at room temperature. Examples of saturated fats are milk, cheese, and meat. These are usually used in making your creamers and whipped toppings. Foods that contain butter, margarine or shortening are also rich in saturated fat. While these are excellent sources of energy, you should keep your consumption of saturated fats to less than 10% of your daily calories. If you consume too much of these products, they tend to deposit in your blood vessels and increase the chances of atherosclerosis. Eating too much saturated fat can increase the amount of cholesterol in your system.

Unsaturated fat is your good fat and are usually liquid at room temperature. You should strive to eat more of your unsaturated fat because these provide you the nutrients needed for body repair and development. Monounsaturated fat is a kind of unsaturated fat that is composed of simpler molecular arrangement. These include your nuts, olives, and avocado. Polyunsaturated fats are composed of fat molecules connected in complex ways. Seafood products are rich in polyunsaturated fats needed by your brain.

The last category of fats is trans-fat. These kinds of foods are highly processed, filled with preservatives and a lot of chemicals that will extend the shelf life of your food. They are also tastier and inviting to eat. Trans-fat can be found in delicious food like your chips, crackers, cookies, and cakes with shortenings. They are very scrumptious, but they are also deadly. They increase the bad cholesterol in your system and may lead to the deposition of fats in your vessels. You should try to minimize the amount of trans-fat you consume daily. They may be very addicting but remember that they will also deal you with a lot of damage in the long run.

The last category of food is your proteins. These are not the main sources of energy. If you exercise, your body will consume your carbohydrates first and your fats next. Only in dire circumstances will your body use up your protein stores. The role of proteins is more of building the body up for growth and strength. Proteins contain a lot of amino acids that are needed for the body to repair itself and to build more cells. Proteins are found mainly in your muscles and skin. Your meat products are excellent sources of proteins as well as some vegetables including your soybeans. You need to maintain a certain amount of protein in your body so you can be physically fit.

The discussion on food may rather be lengthy but these are just the basics of nutrition you need to know. We will discuss more on food on the next chapter. But it is important for you to note the variety of foods and their components. The body will now try to breakdown these foods into simpler components to extract the necessary energy from them.

As you chew your food in your mouth, the food is broken down literally into smaller pieces.

When you swallow, the food enters through your throat and your esophagus, down to your stomach. The stomach is the main digestive area, churning the food and mixing it with acid to break it down further to biochemical pieces. It will enter through your small intestine and this is the area for further digestion but also absorption. The nutrients in the food you ate are now going to be absorbed and carried to the different areas in your body for storage and use. A big component of your food would come from carbohydrates which when broken down, will be reduced to glucose or sugar. It will enter your body from the intestines to your liver and muscles and fat through the blood. When the pancreas sense that there is an increased glucose in the system because of the food intake, it will now release the first hormone, insulin.

The role of insulin is central to our understanding of weight gain. In adults with normal insulin function, the role of insulin is to stimulate your organs to take the glucose or sugar into your fats, muscles and liver and store them for use as energy. The insulin will send messengers to the brain that it is now in a 'fed' state and that the person has enough nutrients so he could stop eating. The muscles, the fats in our body, and the liver will now absorb the glucose from the blood and store it for use as reserved energy. When you do activities such as running or simply moving, your body will be using up the glucose stores. So, because of insulin, that supply is secured. You will now feel subjectively fuller and will stop eating.

Glucagon, on the other hand, is the hormone produced by your body when it senses that there is not enough glucose or energy stored. It is released when the body's energy reserve has been depleted and will signal you to start eating. It puts the body in the 'fasting' state and as a response, you will need to supply your body with food. Your muscles, fats, and liver will be the primary centers for indicating if the energy stores are enough. When you respond to the message of glucagon by eating, then the cycle of insulin-glucagon-insulin-glucagon continues. This is an efficient system of letting your body know when there is enough or not enough food and energy stores to use.

Women with PCOS are very prone to insulin resistance. The exact mechanism of how PCOS and insulin resistance works is not yet very conclusive. But several studies (Norman, et. Al, 2001[7], Teedee, et al, 2006[8]) have already seen the correlation between the two. In insulin resistance, your different organs are not able to recognize insulin and will fail to respond to the call to store glucose. This means that when insulin is released in the blood, your muscles, fats and liver will not sense that insulin is there so it will not reabsorb the glucose. The glucose will stay in your blood and this is measured by glucose strips when you extract blood from a diabetic. There is an elevated degree of glucose in the blood because the muscles, fats and liver are not taking the sugar in and converting it to stored energy. As a result, the muscles, fats and liver will not have enough energy to supply its needs. It will remain the 'fasting' state and will send a signal to your brain to eat more so that you will have more energy. So, you will really gain weight because your system feels that it is not having enough food and energy. Glucagon will also be released as your body is in the 'fasting' state. It will send a signal to your brain to eat more and so you will really binge as a result of the glucagon. Taken together, the deficiency of these two hormones contribute to the feeling of hunger in diabetics and the need to overeat as a result. You will gain more and more weight, but not feel very satisfied with your body and your appetite.

Insulin resistance is only the beginning of the development of Diabetes Mellitus. In insulin resistance, your glucose levels are higher than normal as your muscles, fats and liver are not able to respond to insulin and uptake the glucose. Your body will think that it is fasting. Thus, you are going to see symptoms like eating too much, drinking too much and peeing too much. Your body will feel hungry because there is not enough glucose inside your cells, so you tend to binge. You will feel very dehydrated, so you drink a lot. Because of this excessive drinking, you will also feel the urge to pee most of the time. This triad of symptoms are the beginnings of diabetes mellitus. The diagnosis is mostly through the symptoms you exhibit plus the laboratory findings of elevated glucose in your blood. You have to watch out for diabetes, especially if you have PCOS and/or you have relatives who have diabetes too. Your risk of contracting the disorder increases in these conditions.

If left untreated, your diabetes may not just cost you weight gain, but will target your different organs. People with uncontrolled diabetes may have sickness involving the eyes, the kidneys and nerves. When we talk about the eyes, diabetics have a higher chance of developing cataracts. You may feel blurring of vision and realized that there is a buildup of glucose in your eyes that may cause you to go blind. In terms of your kidney, the glucose may damage your filtration system. You will be peeing out more glucose, which is relatively a heavy and big substance. Through time, the kidneys may be damaged as a result of persistent filtration. This can cause edema or pooling of fluids in your body, pulmonary or coronary diseases. And last, too much glucose will damage your nerves starting from your extremities. The symptoms are often insidious as though you don't feel anything. You may hit a nail and not notice that you stepped on one. It is only when you really observe your foot that you will notice poor wound healing and less sensation in the area. If you don't observe these small accidents, you may result into a diabetic foot, that state where the bacteria from an infected wound may totally eat up your foot and you won't feel anything. This can ultimately ascend further to the knee and to the leg and may require amputation. I am not scaring just for the sake of being a doomsday prophet. I am simply warning of the dire consequences of not controlling your diet and your glucose levels. As a woman with PCOS, I think we have to be extra vigilant regarding our health because we have nature working against us. Insulin resistance and diabetes are warning signs that we have to be more conscious and take active measures.

Chapter 6

The PCOS Diet

One of the pillars of treatment in PCOS involves weight loss. As we have seen in the previous chapters, women with PCOS are very prone to insulin resistance, resulting to weight gain and possibly leading to diabetes. We are very much disadvantaged because no matter what we do, our natural disposition is to continue eating and putting on weight on all the most obvious parts such as our bellies, hips, breasts, arms and thighs. A lot of body issues result from years of being overweight, as we don't fit into the social standards of the pretty skinny woman. Through years of neglect, we may even develop cardiovascular conditions such as hypertension and possible heart attacks or strokes as a result of this genetic predisposition. One of the cornerstones then of healing is the imperative to eat well.

I like the phrase 'eating well' more than dieting or even losing weight because of the positivity of the message. Growing up, I was always told to diet by my family and friends, seeing as how shapely I had become. And for a time, I was a sucker for dieting programs which include tipping on the scale on an everyday basis and slipping through a vicious cycle of days of fasting to moments of binging. I was always sad whenever I would diet because I didn't get to eat the foods that I loved such as cookies, cakes and a lot of desserts. I would content myself with a few crackers to last me a whole day. And after days or even weeks on such a diet, I would give up and on the first whiff of baked goodies, I would cave in. The weight that I lost was quickly regained in a few hours of sin. And those moments instilled great guilt feelings on me, as though I wasn't doing what I should be doing. Dieting was literally 'dying in'.

Over the years, I grew tired of standard diet programs that only led me to more misery and more pounds. As I tried to understand my endocrinal issues, I was able to see where the problem lay and how I could address things in a more relaxed way instead of the suicidal, manic attempts some diet programs approach weight loss. I have realized that crash dieting always crashes and that there is no real need for losing ten pounds in a week. I have compiled here the best tips I have learned through years of trying to eat well to combat PCOS.

Count Your Calories

You may have come across many health and fitness programs that start with a rundown of a lot of nutritional equations. Imagine having to do Math just to lose weight! This may be a big hassle for everyone, especially those who are quite averse to computing anything. Or you may be an advocate of just going with the flow, sticking to good foods but not really being obsessive-compulsive about how much calories you eat. But in my experience, not minding what you eat to the calorie level is very irresponsible and lazy. With so many apps on fitness and nutrition, you may opt not even to do the Math and let this work for you. If you simply go with the flow, you will really not notice any considerable change in the way you eat. You can have an idea of how much you lose or gain in a week by tipping the scale. But without calorie counting, you won't be able to know what foods are causing you to gain weight. Not counting calories is like guessing how healthy you want to be and leaving fate to control your body.

It is difficult to count calories at first. The equations may seem daunting, but once you get the hang of it, you will be able to breeze through a simple calculation. If you aren't really up to it, then you can just use free apps online that will do the counting for you. But calorie counting is essential to any program on eating well. You must know how healthy you are at this point, and what is the target health status you should and want to be.

First, the equation is, of course, the BMI. The BMI measures your overall fitness in terms of the proportion of your weight and height. We have introduced the formula to you a few chapters back. But here it is again:

BMI = weight (in kilograms) / height (in meters)^2

Classify whether you are underweight, normal, overweight, obese I, obese II or morbidly obese. The farther you are from the normal range, the more prone you will be to experience many cardiovascular diseases. The goal is really to have a BMI of 18 to 24kg/m2. If you fall within this range, then we can say that your body is in good shape. Those of you who may be thin are not exactly healthy either. You may not be having enough nutrition to fit your body's needs. Hence, target a BMI within the normal range. Have a target weight you want to be in.

Next, be realistic as to when you want to achieve your ideal weight. If you crash diet and try to lose off more than 10kg in a week, this will harm your body more than benefit you. Consult a dietician or a nutritionist for the optimal meal plan and target weight program that will make you lose weight at a healthy pace. Remember that you will have PCOS all your life and that you don't need to lose all your weight all at once. The body will be responsive to your efforts, just go easy on it.

You need to calculate then the minimum number of calories you will need per day. Calories are a measure of energy. Studies have already devised formulas that show how much energy you will need given your body mass index and your level of activity. This minimal number of calories is expressed in the basic metabolic rate. This refers to how much energy your body uses up in a day. You can compute this by using the Katch-McArdle Formula:

Basic Metabolic Rate: $10W + 6.25H - 5A - 161$

Where,

W is your weight in kilograms

H is your height in centimeters

A is your age

Suppose that a 35-year-old woman who weighs 80 kilograms and has a height of 170cm. What is her basic metabolic rate?

$$BMR = 10\,(80) + 6.25(170) - 5(35) - 161$$

$$= 1,526.5 \text{ calories per day.}$$

We can say that this woman will have to consume 1,526.5 calories per day to maintain her energy requirements. But to this equation, we still have to multiply the activity factor. This factor refers to the level of activity a person usually has in a day.

Activity level factor has the following scores:

Activity	Activity Factor
Sitting/lying down all-day	1.2
Seated work, no exercise	1.3
Seated work, light work	1.4
Moderate physical work, no exercise	1.5
Moderate physical work, light exercise	1.6
Moderate physical work, heavy exercise	1.7
Heavy work/heavy exercise	1.8
Above average physical work/exercise	2.0-2.4

So, if the woman has no work and prefers to lie down all day, her activity factor is 1.2. We multiply that to her basic metabolic rate to get

1,831.8. This is her real caloric daily requirement given the activity level she has on an everyday basis.

Your goal then is to cut down on that daily number of calories slowly so that you lose weight. Again, I repeat that you don't have to overdo the dieting. It is better if you consult a nutritionist and a physician to monitor your weight loss. If you want to lose 1 pound each week, you can opt to decrease your daily caloric need by 500 calories.

Once you obtain the number of calories you will need per week, you will need the help of calorie equivalents. There are countless charts out there which shows how much calories each food has.

For example:

- 8 ounces of sirloin steak (about a fistful) is equivalent to 427 calories
- 1 plain bagel is equivalent to 320 calories
- 1 glass of whole milk is equivalent to 157 calories
- 1 large egg is equivalent to 70 calories

- 1 medium-sized apple is equivalent to 81 calories

Total all the food that you eat in a day and convert them into calories. This is rather tricky because you need to estimate food sizes using portions. Rice is measured in cups for example, or meat in how many fists it covers, etc. The total number of calories from all the foods you eat should not go beyond the total daily caloric requirement you have. If your intent is losing weight, then all the more should you maintain a lower daily requirement. You also have to note all the food preparations you added. Oil, butter and soy sauce all have caloric content. So, everything you eat should be computed and should add up to the daily requirement.

You may find this process very tedious. But this is the only way you can be disciplined in terms of food intake. This is a better method of estimating food intake instead of just guessing how much you eat. Also, calorie counting should not be restrictive.

You have a total target caloric requirement per day. You are free to choose whichever foods you want that will still meet that requirement. If you want to eat sirloin steak today, by all means, order one. But that also means that you have to cut down on the other meals for the rest of the day. Calorie counting is tedious at first, but it will soon pay off in terms of weight loss.

Know Your Carbohydrates and Fats

There are kinds of foods that are 'better' and 'worse' than the others. The 'better' and 'worse' categories only refer to how nutritional important they are in terms of the ease of being digested, energy or caloric content and the harmful side effects they may contain. The basis of these categories is largely from the molecular structure of these foods and how the body digests and absorbs them. A common observation is that most of the 'worse' foods in this list are the tastier and more accessible kinds of foods in the grocery. They are more 'sinful' precisely because they taste so good and yet deal a lot of damage to your system.

In terms of carbohydrates, we were able to note of simple and complex sugars. The general principle is that refined carbohydrates are bad because they are stripped away of nutrition and are easily digested, absorbed and retained in the body. You should decrease your intake of these refined carbohydrates if you are bent on losing weight. Bad or refined carbohydrates include:

- Fruit juices
- Soda or soft drinks
- Cakes and pastries
- Potato chips and french fries
- White rice or bread

Whole or unprocessed carbohydrates are good because they contain all the natural nutrients in the food. They may be digested and absorbed less quickly than refined sugars, but they provide the same amount of calories or energy you need. You should eat more of the following whole carbohydrates:

- Fresh fruits
- Fresh vegetables
- Beans, lentils, peas
- Whole grains
- Brown rice
- Seeds (pumpkin, quinoa, chia)
- Sweet potatoes

In terms of fats, we already discussed the difference between saturated, polyunsaturated, mono-unsaturated and trans-fatty food. We said that we need to decrease the intake of foods high in trans-fatty acid. Increased consumption of trans-fat rich foods will increase the bad cholesterol in your body which leads to the narrowing and eventual blocking of your blood vessels leading to potential stroke or heart attack. In general, lessen your intake of the following foods with high trans-fat content:

- Crackers
- Pizza
- Microwave popcorn

- Coffee creamer
- Fast food (French fries, breaded chicken, etc.)

On the other hand, I recommend that you increase your intake of the polyunsaturated fat foods which aid in your body repair and development. These foods include:

- Salmon
- Sardines
- Nuts (walnuts, peanut, cashew)
- Avocado

Try Vegan

You can never go wrong with eating vegetables. Rich in fiber and a lot of nutrients, vegetables are good sources of nutrition. The fiber in plants is particularly useful for helping in digestion and preventing constipation. They are easily available in markets and may be prepared in a variety of ways. But sadly, a lot of people are still skipping their vegetables because they find it tasteless or unappetizing. Children, in particular, are first introduced to processed food which is tasty. When served with vegetables, their palettes are already craving for the junk food they first tasted. Preparing tasty vegetables is then a challenge for cooks and food handlers.

Also, contrary to popular belief, vegetables also contain the protein you need for your diet. Many people associate chicken, beef, and pork as the only sources of protein. But you can also get your protein from tofu, beans, green peas, sweet corn, artichokes, and broccoli. To reach your recommended protein consumption, you just have to double your servings of these kinds of foods.

Vegetables can be prepared in a variety of ways. They can be steamed, fried, baked, blanched, grilled, sautéed, puréed, curried, or pickled. Explore ways of how you can experiment with vegetables so it can be appetizing for you and for the people you want to cook for. For example, there are recipes which now treat cauliflower as meat. You can now enjoy cauliflower as a hamburger patty. While your veggies may be healthy, the oil they were cooked in may not be. Therefore, I recommend using avocado or olive oil when cooking. If you want to really adopt a healthy lifestyle, be conscious of all the things that you put in your food.

Include Herbs and Essential Oils

There is not a lot of research tackling the use of essential oils and herbs to treat PCOS. To start off, these oils are extracted from plants by means of physical pressing or steaming. The oil that is taken from these processes are the ones commercially packaged and sold in stores. Note that oils should always be from natural resources and not chemically made. With so much of these oils around, it is a pity not many are looking to unlock how these can be used to help alleviate the symptoms of PCOS. It is not clear if the use of essential oils alone helps PCOS or if it is able to induce healing together with other medications. I have come across some researches but most of these covered only a limited population. Hence, the use of essential oils is not yet conclusive. You may opt to use these at your own risk. I will tackle some of these only in so far as some research has been done on their benefit on PCOS.

Clary Sage

More commonly found in the Northern Mediterranean area, clary sage has been traditionally used as a medicinal plant. It is usually inhaled which means you burn the oil and take in the scent of the oil for aromatherapy. The smell of clary sage is said to bring about a state of calmness and boosts the mood of people. This is helpful in terms of warding off the stress that can trigger your hormonal imbalance. There are some who say that inhaling clary sage can balance estrogen levels in women with PCOS, improving symptoms related to vaginal bleeding. Though this is not clinically proven, the use of the oil outweighs the harm it can do.

Thyme

More commonly used in cooking and roasting of meat dishes, thyme can also be used as an essential oil. The use of thyme has been linked to improve the progesterone levels of women with PCOS. Remember that without follicle-stimulating hormone, there is no induction of ovulation and no production of progesterone. With the use of thyme oil, progesterone levels are induced, helping in the ovulation of a woman. The use of thyme may also be beneficial to balance out mood swings and hot flashes as encountered in menopause. It has also been found to induce weight loss in some cases.

Spearmint

A study by Ataabadi, et al (2017[9]) had explored the use of spearmint to combat hirsutism and acne in women. Spearmint was found to have anti-androgenic properties. The study was conducted on mice who were given different amounts of spearmint oil. Results showed that mice who were given spearmint oil had reduced weight, decreased testosterone levels and increased follicular development. Though not yet applied to women with PCOS, this study shows the promising potential of spearmint to decrease symptoms of PCOS. By simply applying spearmint oil in our body, we may be able to minimize hair excess, acne, and weight gain.

There are many other essential oils that are being studied in relation to their benefits to alleviating PCOS. I am surprised that the use of essential oils is not as common as pharmaceutical medications in treating this condition. The potential of essential oils is not maximized when we don't explore ways of how to use these naturally occurring substances.

Small, Frequent Meals

One way you can trick your body to feel full without binging is to eat small but frequent meals. An average person eats around 3-4 meals a day, assuming that each meal is a full meal. For breakfast, you can have avocado and egg which is a good combination of fat and protein. For lunch, you can have chicken, pork or beef, with a side of vegetables. Dinner would probably be the same as lunch. And then you can have snacks in between meals, like nuts. It looks pretty balanced because you are working in between meals. When you eat breakfast, your work afterward until lunchtime. From lunch, you resume work until you are hungry enough for dinner. And then there is the long fast until you break it in breakfast. The cycle repeats.

Your body may be accustomed to this rhythm of feeding. But this is not the only way your body can feel nourished. In fact, there are other ways that will give a subjective feeling of fullness, but not necessarily a lot to increase your weight. One such method is the small but frequent meals method. In this meal plan, the normal 3 major meals and 2 snacks are broken down to 8 small meals throughout the day. Try dividing your waking hours into 8. This means that you will be eating one meal every one and half to two hours. But to compensate for the frequency, the portion of servings is also reduced. Instead of having one big hefty breakfast, imagine eating the same thing at two different intervals. You can have egg at 7 AM and then an avocado at 8:30 AM. By using this method, the body will not feel hungry throughout the day because you are eating more frequently. But you are not gaining more weight because the servings per meal should actually be less than if you eat three full meals.

Whenever you eat a big amount of food, a large amount of insulin is released in response to the influx of glucose. The amount of hormones produced is proportional to the amount of food needed to be consumed. If you eat small meals, the pancreas would not be as stressed because there is less food to digest. Our digestive organs can handle smaller pieces compared to big boluses on regular intervals. Also, when we skip meals in a three-meal-setup, there is a tendency to overeat to compensate for the lost food intake. The big meal intake would then require the stomach and pancreas to secrete more acids and hormones. If you skip meals often, the lining of your stomach and your intestines may be damaged in the future. When you eat the eight food servings per day, your body will really feel full from the increased frequency of feeding. The body won't even notice if the calories are halved. By using the small but frequent meals method, you will be able to slowly lose your weight without the struggle of dying from dieting.

Chapter 7

Managing Weight

When you plan to lose weight, eating well must be supplemented with good activity. Remember that your body is not made to store energy, but to use it well. You may be eating the right kind of food, but with a sedentary, couch potato lifestyle, your gains may be arrested. The next pillar of healing PCOS is through a good amount of exercise. We need to use all those energies in building up our bodies. You don't need to have abs or sculpted physique just to say that you are healthy and beautiful. Those might look nice and are often the dream bodies of most women. But my personal experience tells me that having a body where you are able to function well and independently, able to perform various tasks with ease, comfortable to move around is enough. You are beautiful when your body is able to be at its optimal best. I believe that you can be in any body shape or size as long as you are able to do the various activities of the day with ease. If you are heaving and puffing from simply walking around in your own weight, I don't think that is healthy. We can all do our part in sweating out once in a while.

Many people will often skip this part for a number of reasons. Some find fitness programs and gym memberships expensive. Others aren't willing to invest in exercise equipment for lack of money, time or space. The ultimate excuse, of course, is that people don't have time to exercise. They lead so very busy lives on a 24-hour shift, from putting in the work at the office, attending to various meetings, performing various errands, attending to family, socializing and commuting. But if you look closely at their lifestyle, they are still able to go about drinking to the wee hours or more or spending as much as 4 hours on social media. If you think you are too busy to exercise, then you must be leading an unhealthy kind of busy. It is a problem of laziness, a problem of wrong priorities, and a problem of weak willpower. Here are some tips I have in boosting your will to be fit and have an active lifestyle.

Start a Routine

The most effective way to start anything new is to incorporate it into a routine. You will find it much easier if you don't have to think about what to do on a regular day because you have set a daily schedule. The trick really lies in training the brain to anticipate the same things in an unpredictable course of activities. Schedule your sleep time and wake up time. If you are comfortable waking up at 7 AM, then set your alarm for 7 AM and practice waking at the same time every day. Next, be faithful to your mealtimes. Eat regular breakfast, lunch, and dinner. Part of the routine is training your stomach to anticipate mealtimes on a regular basis. Lastly, schedule your activities in the morning, the afternoon and the evening. You might have a lot of variations given your dynamic work. But at least you have set the work hours to a fixed time. There may be times where you may be required to stay later at work. Keep these at a minimum. You are not being paid to work extra-long. The work hours are set because the company has measured that the highest productivity is only within a certain amount of time. Your weekends can then be more variable. This is an area where you can be creative and try out different things. After the weekend is over, embrace the rhythm of the new week once again.

You may already have a certain routine developed already. This time, try looking for dead spaces in your schedule where you can put in at least 30 minutes of exercise thrice a week. Exert an effort to squeeze in some time for physical activity. If you only sit down and really analyze your week, you will find spare time for a quick run or an exercise routine. If you really value a healthy body, then you can give priority to exercising. Think of activities in your week you can give up or cut back so that you can spend some time developing your body.

The golden period to develop any habit is three weeks. If you want to train your body to work in a particular way, you should be doing the same activities for 21 days. The first week will be very difficult as you are adjusting to the new schedule. You may miss some set events or linger on a few tasks once in a while. But try as much as possible to be religious in sticking to your daily regimen. Once you get a hang of it, you will find that your body will be craving for the boring monotony of routine. It is as if the body wants to control the anticipation of activities. After three weeks, you may go on auto-pilot mode and your body is set to follow your schedule. You won't have trouble pushing yourself to go to the gym or attend your yoga session because your body is already used to it and will welcome the tension.

Walk and Take the Stairs

The point in exercise is to let the blood circulate in your system. If you review the city living lifestyle, many of us lead sedentary lives. If you only try to clock in every activity for every hour, you will be surprised to find out that you spend most of your day in front of a computer or a mobile phone. From the moment you wake up to the moment before you sleep, the first thing you grab is your phone. You spend some minutes checking out messages on your social media and update yourself with the world. Throughout the day, you may think that your phone usage is minimal because you only open your phone occasionally, in between work breaks. But those occasions when taken together can reach as much as 4 to 6 hours of total usage. You don't notice that you have been using your phone for the longest time because it is spread out throughout the day. And then in the office, you may be behind a task, typing away on a keyboard or browsing through a screen in the morning. The next time you put that mouse down, you find out that it is already night outside. And then you may be so tired from all that sitting and brain exertion that you just want to lie down in bed or couch, watching television until you fall asleep.

This is a dangerous lifestyle to lead. Yes, it is comfortable but in the longer run, a sedentary lifestyle will predispose you to a lot of cardiovascular diseases. Remember that food is energy, and the more energy you don't use, these will only deposit in your body as fat. Too much fat deposition may clog up your blood vessels leading to cardiovascular events. When blood is not circulating well, the toxins inside your body are not flushed out efficiently. You also don't deliver as much oxygen as your body needs. You will feel tired more easily and it will be heavier to drag your body to do any physical activity. A sedentary lifestyle will kill you in the longer run.

So, find ways to jolt you out of this bum life. You have to exert extra effort to move your body. The motto should be to move, move, and move! You can accomplish these through a number of ways. Take the stairs instead of riding the elevator. If you live on a very high floor, stop the elevator just halfway through and then walk the rest. Walk instead of taking a cab on short distances. Cook your food instead of ordering to-go. Take time to do manual chores in the house such as gardening, brushing the floor, tidying up space. Jog in place when you are not doing anything. These small acts when taken together have a big impact on your body. You will feel that your blood is circulating better when you are able to breathe easier and you feel lighter. You may be more flexible to move around because of these small bursts of energy.

You will also need to cut down on unnecessary couch potato activities. Of course, you need to use your phone. But try setting a limit to your usage. If you normally use up 5 hours, try using your phone only for 4. The change need not be drastic. There should just be some change in the usual inactive lifestyle. It will be difficult at first. But once you start the habit, you will realize that you can cut down on your phone and computer usage. You can actually do all the things you really need to do at a shorter time if you put an effort into it.

Find an Exercise You Like

Continuing from an active, anti-sedentary lifestyle, you still should find an exercise routine that will work for you. The small bouts of activity in the previous tips are only meant to make you exercise and are not in themselves, substitute for the real thing. You still have to allot a specific time to work out.

The goal should not be to have abs or a sculpted body. While that may be ideal and motivating for young people, it may not be realistic for those who are well into their adult and menopausal years. Your body ages too and if you push yourself with too much exercise, your body might not be able to handle it. There is such a thing as over-exercising, and you may damage your body more if you exhaust it. The goal is really to find an activity that will help you sweat for at least 30 minutes three times a week.

With this condition, walking leisurely then is not considered exercise. You may spend two hours walking or shopping along a busy street and feel tired. But if you didn't sweat, then it is not an exercise. If you do rapid walking for at least 30 minutes and you can feel both exhaustion and perspiration, then you have accomplished your goal.

I can't recommend any particular exercise program that you should indulge in. I am of the opinion that you should be doing an activity that you like and that will make you sweat. If you are a gym type of person, then the gym is for you. If you are more into yoga and flexibility rather than weight training, then that is also acceptable. You may find biking a thrill or rowing as a new sport. By all means, explore all the kinds of activities that will keep you moving. The point here is to do something that will make you happy and sweaty. If you don't like going to the gym, you will only feel forced to do it. Exercising then will become a chore for you, another one of the musts that you have no choice but to do. This will eventually tire you out and sooner or later, you'd drop out of your program. But if you enjoy the kind of exercise you chose, the physical activity will not be a chore for you, but a form of release you may crave for.

Exercise does not only aid in circulation. When you move, you are also stimulating your endorphins, the pleasure hormone in the brain. Endorphins will activate your reward center. When they are released, you will feel happy and satisfied. The endorphins pathway in your brain may also be stimulated when you do something pleasurable such as eating chocolate, hugging and kissing your loved ones or having a relaxing massage. When you exercise, your body will feel very relaxed and pleasurable. This will give you more incentive then to exercise.

I recommend having only thirty minutes of exercise three times a week. This is enough time to help the blood circulate in your body and keep your muscles strong. Be wary of exhausting yourself by over-exercising. Instead of feeling pleasure, you may feel pain and aches all over. You may even damage connective tissues and fatigue your muscles. So do things only in moderation. Exercise some and keep your energy flowing. Your exercise may even benefit other parts of your life such as being productive at work. Being physically healthy will not only be for your benefit. Your health will also benefit others.

Join a Club

We also have to introduce the concept of exercising with others. While you may be so motivated about exercising, it can be quite lonely at times. Imagine lifting weights alone on the gym, with no one but you looking at the mirror. You will do feel your muscles flexing and the strain of the weights on your shoulders and arms. But it isn't as enjoyable as exercising with others.

There are actually studies that show how exercising with others can actually boost efficiency. Even the mere presence of other people around you can develop a sense of competition, as though you are trying to edge out the others. This mini competition may drive you to run one more mile, to swim faster, to hold on a yoga pose a minute longer, to lift 2kgs more of weights. A study by the Rackow (2015)[10] shows us that having an exercise buddy or partner increased the gym going activities of participants. She asked one group of participants to find an exercise buddy and the other half to continue exercising. Her research showed that the first group were more faithful to their gym schedule and exercised more consistently than those without an exercise buddy. This supports the idea that you will experience more endorphins when you exercise with others.

Friendships can also develop when you join an exercise club. Your social network is expanded while you are improving your own body. This can provide you with the social support you may need to keep you motivated to keep healthy. When you gain friends in the gym or while running, your newfound friends can keep you exercising as they will look out for you. There may be times when you don't feel like exercising, but your friends can pull you out of your lazy streak. The feeling is actually more heightened when many people are working towards keeping themselves fit and healthy, inside of a one-woman ascent to health. The load seems lighter when you exercise together.

Sleep

Finally, one of the most important, but often neglected, aspects of health is sleep. When you really want to be healthy, you should get enough sleep. In our quest to become successful in our career, we often trade sleep for a few more hours of productive work, one last page to type, and one last presentation slide to perfect. We think that we can just get back the sleep we lost in a night by snatching some hours during the day. We may eat the healthiest foods and be religious in our exercise regimen, but without sleep, you will still feel unhealthy.

Sleep has many important functions that are essential to our development. Sleep provides us with rest, both in our mind and in our bodies. You may be working so hard during the day. Sleep will give you back the strength you need so you can work more the next day. If you don't get enough sleep, your muscles and organs can be prone to damage due to overuse. Like an engine, your body can overheat when you don't give it the rest it deserves.

Sleep also consolidates learning. When you sleep, the mind rearranges itself to synthesize all the data it has received during the day. So, it is not actually effective when you are studying late at night and cramming all the information in your head without sleeping. You need to sleep so that your brain can process everything and solidify the learning. You are actually going to be less productive when you don't sleep as you are prone to errors and inattention. Little important details can be overlooked because you are not concentrating enough due to lack of sleep. Even a few hours of quality sleep can actually boost your memory and make you more efficient.

Since PCOS involves a lot of hormones, sleep will also be very beneficial to your endocrinal system. There are certain hormones like your growth, melatonin and gonadotropin hormones (for reproduction) that are secreted only when you sleep and when the environment is dark. Lack of sleep can actually contribute to your PCOS, messing up with your hypothalamus-pituitary-ovarian axis. Your PCOS may actually worsen because your endocrines are very sensitive to darkness and a state of rest.

How much sleep then is enough? Is 15 minutes alright or do we need 10 hours of sleep? The average quality of sleep is around 7-9 hours for adult according to the National Sleep Foundation[11]. But the actual number of hours you need will actually depend on you. There are people who only have 4 hours of sleep but feel rested afterward. There are people who sleep for 10 hours straight but feel very tired after. The point of sleep is to induce a state of restfulness. You will need to gauge how much sleep you need to make you feel rested. Another thing is that you cannot just buy back the sleep you lost in the night for sleeping in the day. When you don't sleep at night, those are hours of sleep lost forever. You are not going to feel rested by always sleeping during the day. The best sleep is still at night so make sure that you stick to a regular schedule. Sleep well and your body will be more optimal.

Chapter 8

Think Positively

One of the most neglected aspect in understanding PCOS is mental health. Medicine has grossly focused on the mechanisms of PCOS and how it brings about various endocrinal abnormalities. Medications on PCOS are all targeted at increasing fertility, managing acne or hair excess. But these measures largely ignore the psychological impact of all these changes in women. Some even brush off mental issues of women with PCOS as a case of overreacting or women's emotional whims. Others are bullied into silence, thinking that their issues are to be ashamed of. The mental health of women with PCOS is largely an unwritten history, with women forced to accept their condition in silence. PCOS should not stress you because stress might be one of the reasons you are not getting better.

Living with PCOS, I did go through some rather dark days. Growing up, I used to feel ugly about how I looked. I was fat, pimply and hairy as a teenage girl and I suffered through that. School was a rather bittersweet experience. On the one hand, I had a lot of bullies trying to trip me or throw my bag on the trash can, all for not looking good. But on the other, I was able to channel that sadness into academics and I excelled well. When I reached my twenties, I thought I was past those pubertal scars. But the weight gain simply never stopped. There were days when I didn't want to go out. There was a very dark point when I even thought of ending it all.

But the moment I met a friend in college who also had PCOS, my world changed completely. I didn't know other people had PCOS. I was researching about the subject when my roommate saw what I was browsing. Out of the blue, she told me she had PCOS too. And that was the start of a long friendship. We traded a lot of sob stories of being bullied and not getting the guys we wanted. We would often eat out together and eating didn't feel as guilty anymore. As I listened to her stories, I felt that I was not alone in my struggle. She was my savior and I was able to get through the rest of college and adulthood because of her.

The more I became focused on my interest in PCOS, I began to interview a lot more women. I realized that there were really a lot of women with PCOS, but they just weren't talking about it. I heard a lot of stories of bad relationships, anxiety attacks, and depressive episodes. I cried with them as we recalled traumatic experiences of being rejected. And after hearing these stories, I vowed to chronicle their struggles. PCOS is not just a medical issue. It is a condition that affects our minds and perhaps, that is the worst part of it.

In my interviews, I realized that women with PCOS are prone to a host of mental issues. The most prominent of these are anxiety and depression. These conditions may coexist with PCOS, are reinforced by it and even aggravate PCOS. Women are not diagnosed to have these conditions because they don't seek any help. They don't even see that anxiety and depression are real problems that are treatable. They will only seek help when they have reached the worse. For some, their depression and anxiety have led them to a point of no return. And this is sad and should be stopped.

Anxiety is defined as the feeling of unease over an anticipated event. Women with PCOS often have anxiety when they are meeting other people, speaking in front of a crowd, socializing with strangers, catching up during reunion. Much of the anxiety has been reinforced over past experiences, starting from childhood. Into their adulthood, they carry these traumas and feel anxious. But much of the anxiety is only in the mind. The thing they are anxious about may be real or imagined. For example, the woman with PCOS may be very anxious upon attending a high school reunion. She fears that her classmates will bring back ugly memories of her and will now compare how they are successful in the present. This may be both true and false. Perhaps, her friends will really bring it up. Or perhaps, the topics will not even be remotely about her. But in her mind, the anxious woman is convinced she is going to be a victim. And so, she doesn't attend.

We all feel anxiety at times. Anxiety is a normal feeling in response to the unknown. But it becomes pathological when there is already a loss of social functions as a result of the anxiety. The clinical diagnosis of anxiety on adults[12] should cover several symptoms observed on a person over 6 months. There should be the presence of excessive anxiety with at least three of the following: edginess or restlessness, easy fatigability, impaired concentration, irritability, increased muscle aches, and difficulty sleeping. When you observe someone or yourself to have these, then it may be time to seek a consult.

Depression goes hand in hand with anxiety. It is an extreme form of sadness. As such, we can say that sadness covers a broad spectrum of emotions. You can be mildly irritated. You can be moping, or demoralized. You can be grieving or mortified. And on the extreme, you can be depressed. When you have reached this lowest point, it is important for you to seek help.

Women with PCOS are prone to depression because of three mechanisms. One, they think they are bad and unworthy because of their appearance and their incapacity. Second, they think that their environment is bad, that their friends, family and total strangers are out to judge them. And third, they think that there is no hope for the future to get better. This triad of negative thinking reinforce each other and the woman with PCOS finds herself being pulled down into an endless spiral of depression.

The clinical diagnosis of depression is made on an adult patient over a minimum of 2 weeks observation span. There should be a depressed move or loss of interest or pleasure plus five or more of the following symptoms: significant weight loss or loss of appetite, slowing down of thought, easy fatigability, feeling of worthlessness or guilt, inability to concentrate, recurring thoughts of death or suicide. If you spot some of these on a person, alert them to immediately seek help.

What should we do once we get wind of some of these symptoms? You may not see all of them immediately, but even just a few should already alarm you to observe the person more closely. We do not want very extreme situations where the woman with PCOS is pushed to suicide ideation or actual attempt because of these negative thoughts. Here are some of my tips in boosting our mental health.

Recognize the Problem and Seek Help

In all self-development programs such as for alcoholic or drug users, the very first step to the process of healing is the recognition that you have a problem. There can be no healing if there is no first acceptance of one's condition. Some people's reaction to a mental condition is to deny that they have a problem. Women with PCOS may claim that their anxiety is normal, or that it is part of their monthly mood swings. They try to defend themselves with all sorts of rationale why they act the way they do. And this is very counterproductive. One, it delays any sort of intervention. If you deny that you have a problem, then it will take you longer to seek any help, much less get treated. You may only seek help when you are really into deep and often irreversible problems already. Second, the real issue is not being addressed. You may often blame your faulty menstrual cycle for all the troubles you are experiencing. By putting the fault on another person or issue, you are evading responsibility for it. You don't accept that you are capable of being weak as well. And because of this, your mental health issues will continue to aggravate deep within until it just explodes.

We are weak and vulnerable. We should accept that as women with PCOS, we are limited. Yes, you have a stellar education and a good career. You may hold a high position in your company, and you may have a lot of achievements in life. But you are not also invincible. You are not perfect, no matter how hard you try to be. And it's ok. It is ok to be not ok sometimes. It's perfectly fine if you make a few mistakes here and there. It is ok if you don't get the promotion you've longed for. It's ok if you can't have a child after many years of trying. It's ok. We don't need to be perfect for anyone. We just have to be real to ourselves and to others.

It takes courage to accept that we have a disorder. It is hard to reconcile the fact that in spite of our achievements, we still need help sometimes. It can be humiliating at times when we realize how weak we really are. But once you have reached this bottom, you can only go up from now on. Once you recognize that you have a problem and that you need somebody's help, the healing is already taking place. It is shameful at first, but once you've accepted who you are, faults and gifts together, you are opening yourself to the possibility of being cured.

Seek help because there are a lot of resources out there that will aid in your healing. You might think that psychiatrist and therapists are only for the crazy. But what's normal anyway? Perhaps, we are all some kind of crazy and thus we need professionals who may be in the best position to process our thoughts and feelings. By seeking professional help, you are entrusting your secrets and vulnerabilities to one person who has studied his or her life to help you in your condition. Medication is but one of the many ways we heal. But even the mere telling of your story to another person is already healing in itself. A hug from a friend, a call from someone you have not heard of for a long time, a smile from your partner may be all you need to go through every rough day.

Find Your Support Group

You are not alone. Some may even have problems way worse than you. For you PCOS may be the end of the world, but for the one sitting beside you, being unable to become pregnant may be a torture. When you join a support group, it may be awkward at first to open to complete strangers. But when people start opening up their own fears and anxieties, it is like a reunion of friends facing the same darkness. By listening to how others are also as weak and vulnerable as you are, you will feel that the burden does not need to be shouldered alone. Your weakness is also your strength because it is through it that you can relate to other women who are also hurt.

Sometimes, it is hard to talk to a male doctor when they talk about endocrinal abnormalities of PCOS. I used to have a male endocrinologist explaining to me how my menstrual system works. He covered all the textbook points throughout his discussion. But I just felt empty listening to his medical jargon. I would clam up when he would ask me if I had questions. I just didn't know if I could trust him with stupid questions like "why can't I have babies with my partner?' or 'when is the best time to try having sex?'. Maybe I was too harsh and judgmental, but it was hard to open up to him. When he would lecture over the connection of my hypothalamus to my pituitary to my ovary, I didn't know if he could even feel the pain inside when all these happen.

But when you open up to somebody who has gone through the roughest times with PCOS, then there is a sense of kinship. I had an easier time believing other women with PCOS because I know that they were undergoing similar experiences as I am. And so, this is my message to you. I know what you are going through and I am with you. We can triumph over PCOS together. You don't even have to pretend to be strong every day. You don't have to put on a fake smile and say you are ok to every person concerned about your health. I've been through the same things as you, and I am here to experience this rollercoaster of feelings with you. But you must allow another person in, before all the healing can happen. By joining a support group, you are allowing other people to share the burden with you.

Be Thankful

Start each day with gratitude for three things. You can be as specific as you want to be. You can be thankful for waking you up in the morning. You can be thankful for having three meals a day. You can be thankful for the comfortable bed you slept in last night. It may be hard at first to name three things you are grateful for each day. But if you really put an effort to remembering your day and thinking of three things you are most grateful for, you will realize that there are actually a lot.

Gratitude is the antidote to depression. Yes, there is the standard medications to combat depression such as your sleeping pills or your anti-anxiety pills or your uppers. But the less costly and more effective cure to depression is to keep being grateful every day. What does it even mean to be grateful?

There are three things to remember in gratitude: the gift, the giver and the present. These are very interrelated words which we would dwell on. First, the gift is the primary reason we are being grateful. The gift is the source of our happiness. When we receive a toy during Christmas, we are overwhelmed with joy. When you receive a fat paycheck, an anniversary ring or good news from your parents, then that object fills you up with such joy. Gifts are always sources of happiness that is why we look forward to receiving gifts. When we are depressed, we are just drained from all the joy in the world. In our self-pity, we fail to recognize that there are a lot of gifts around us. We fail to seek joy in the simple things surrounding us. When you are too sad, you fail to see how the weather is actually pleasant, or that the secretary greeted you or the cook made your dish extra special. We are so wrapped up in our own sadness that we cannot be surprised with simple joys. That is why we need to exert an effort to be grateful.

Second, more than the gift, we should also be focusing on the giver. That Christmas toy did not just pop from nowhere; it might have been Santa Claus, but my guess is that it would have been your parents who love you very much. That promotion and paycheck came from a boss or the company that trusts and approves of your work and the value you put in. That anniversary ring was given by your partner as a sign of his love. All of our gifts come from another person. When we are grateful, we recognize someone that is giving us the gift. We recognize that there are other people who love us and care for us genuinely. When we are depressed, we can only think about ourselves. When we are depressed, it is all about me, me and me. When we are grateful, that 'me' fades in the background of the generosity of others. You will see just how big the world is beyond your selfish imagination. And this world is not out there to judge you. Yes, there will be mean people who will bully you but not everyone. I will not judge you. And there are a lot of people who will accept you for who you are. This is only possible if you let other people gift you with their love.

And finally, the gifts from the giver are given in the present. I like that wordplay between gifts and present. They both pertain to an object of blessing and love. But another dimension of present is the time element. You are being gifted now. You are being showered with love now. You are blessed in the present. When you try to do the gratitude exercise, you are recalling all the gifts you have received in the present day. And it is very important to dwell in the present. When you are anxious or depressed, your mind is only preoccupied with two things: the past and the future. You worry about the past and are saddened by your experiences. You worry about the future, how everyone will judge you, how you will be miserable, how much money you need to finance your medication. And this preoccupation with the past and the present will only make you feel more anxious and depressed. When you are grateful, you leave the past and the future away for a time. The past is already past, and there is nothing you can change about it. The future is not yet here and so why worry about it. But you have to stay in the present and derive joy just being in this moment. This second will pass away very quickly. So, keep on relishing the present because that in itself is a gift you can find joy in.

Keep a Journal

I find writing one of the most therapeutic ways to calm myself whenever I feel panicky or depressed. I didn't write journals before because I found it too tedious to maintain. But when my therapist suggested that I write, I was surprised at how I naturally picked up the pace. There is something about writing that is calming. I suppose it is the manual writing of letters which can be slow at times compared to the thoughts in mind. My mind can be racing with so many thoughts that I couldn't focus. But when I write, I am forced to concentrate on only one thought at a time. I am able to trim down what I really want to say out of the chaos of feelings running through me. There is an order in writing, something I also wanted to experience in my personal life.

And this is also my advice to you. Keep a journal of your daily life. Chronicle what you are feeling on a particular day, what were your activities, what were the thoughts you had, who were the people you were dealing with. Write without too much filtering because at the end of the day, you are the only one who is going to read it. Don't try to impress anyone with your style of writing or the creative content of your activities. Just be yourself. If your day was boring, just write how boring it is. If you feel anxious, write down the things that make you feel panicky. If you are depressed, write down the things that make you sad. If a lot of things happened in your day, focus on one that really struck you the most. If you are not used to writing, you may find the exercise difficult. You may think that you don't have anything important enough to write. But if you just make an effort, your thoughts and feelings will just flow into your journal. There is too much happening in your life that a journal cannot contain.

And it's wonderful to read a journal after completing months' or years' worth of entries. You will really see progress in the kind of person you are when you started writing compared to the person you have become now. When you journal, you are able to trace the development of mood swings and feelings, how you have been anxious at the simplest things or how you got through difficult challenges. Your journal chronicles the healing process you have undergone. And it is important to remember all these changes. You may be able to learn lessons on how you were able to cope with past stressors by rereading your journal. You can thank specific people who have helped you along your journey. With writing and reading journals, you will be able to make sense of your life purpose. Perhaps, you had to go through those rough times to make you the strong person you are now. I believe that there is no accident and that you are exactly in the place you are meant to be now. If you are finding life difficult now, perhaps it is because you have to learn something from it now that will enable you to be happy in the future. Your journal will be with you, telling your story of healing. And if you are open enough, maybe you can even let others read your journal so that they can be inspired too.

Love Yourself

One of the most neglected aspects of healing in PCOS is self-care. There is so much preoccupation with medication and surgical treatments, but it really boils down to loving yourself as a crucial step in healing yourself. Women with PCOS, in their quest to be rid of the symptoms of PCOS, neglect to take time and appreciate their own beauty. They listen most of the time to what others will say or what media will dictate as the standard of beauty and health. And they only get anxious and depressed over these messages. Instead of seeking love from other people, please give it to yourself first.

Find something that you enjoy doing. If you really like painting but haven't gotten the time, take a break from work and get those brushes out. If you love traveling, then a change of scenery will do wonders for you. Buy those shoes you've always wanted. Take that extreme sport you've only imagined doing. Find that place you've always dreamt of going to. Or just take time out to sleep and chill for a while, nothing dramatic. Whatever it is, you need to start taking care of yourself. This is not being selfish. It is about caring for yourself first so that you can care for others more fully. If you are used to minding the concerns of other people, then you may be neglecting your own. And most of the time, we don't feel as appreciated or as valued as we thought we deserve. Instead of waiting for that "Thank you" or "You are intelligent all along" comments, start loving yourself today.

Try looking at yourself in the mirror. Concentrate on each body part. Look at your body from head to foot, from left to right, at all angles. Look at all the unwanted spots you have. Look at the curves in your body. Can you say that you are beautiful? If you cannot say that, then don't expect other people will say that to you. There must be first an acceptance of your unique beauty before others can notice it. You are beautiful, no matter who you are. Yes, we may be shapely. Yes, we may have a lot of hair and acne. Yes, we may be moody at times. But that is what we are. And these make us all the more beautiful. Say that repeatedly to yourself, "I am beautiful, inside and out." This mantra, when repeated, becomes part of you. Even if you don't feel like it, by repeating it over and over, you are going to feel like it and even look the part. This inner glow is the start of a beauty manifesting itself from inside out. You are beautiful as you are. Believe and continue to flourish.

Conclusion

Having lived with PCOS all my life, I have experienced all the ups and downs in moods, feelings and thoughts. More than the endocrinal abnormalities happening inside me, I felt that the psychological and social stigma of PCOS greatly added to the burden of living with this condition. I have seen how PCOS can bring out the worst in me in terms of my work, my relationships, and my love for myself. I have also seen how people react towards me as I went through different transitional stages. And after many years of fighting with PCOS, I was able to achieve a certain peace with this disorder. I still have PCOS and will still have PCOS until I die. But that thought does not scare me or even worry me the least bit. I have learned through years of experience, research, and conversations with other women with PCOS that PCOS is only as powerful in controlling your life as you want it to be. This means that you have the actual power over PCOS. You have the capacity to understand it and how it affects your systems. By knowledge, you may have reached a certain control of how much your body is already affected by PCOS. You also have the power to manage it. PCOS is a lifelong condition, but it can be treated with proper diet, exercise, and positive thinking.

These are the only keywords you need to live by and be at peace with PCOS. These words have guided me through these years and I have been preaching these simple steps to other women with PCOS who are still afraid, lost and anxious. I see them still letting PCOS take control of their lives instead of the other way around. And so, I hope that by reading this book, you take that power from PCOS and restore it for yourself. Share these as well with other women and together, we can build a community of empowered PCOS survivors. In medicine, the acronym PCOS stands for 'polycystic ovarian syndrome.' But for me, I will remember it as 'Persons Choosing to Own Salvation'. The disorder does not hold power over us. We are more powerful and beautiful than our condition.

References

[1] Center for Disease Control and Prevention. *PCOS (Polycystic Ovarian Syndrome and Diabetes.* Retrieved from https://www.cdc.gov/diabetes/basics/pcos.html

[2] Hoffman, B. L., & Williams, J. W. (2012). *Williams gynecology.* New York: McGraw-Hill Medical.

[3] Hoffman, B. L., & Williams, J. W. (2012). *Williams gynecology.* New York: McGraw-Hill Medical.

[4] World Health Organization. (2020) *Body Mass Index.* Retrieved from http://www.euro.who.int/en/health-topics/disease-prevention/nutrition/a-healthy-lifestyle/body-mass-index-bmi

[5] Hoffman, B. L., & Williams, J. W. (2012). *Williams gynecology.* New York: McGraw-Hill Medical.

[6] Hoffman, B. L., & Williams, J. W. (2012). *Williams gynecology*. New York: McGraw-Hill Medical.

[7] Norman, R. J., Masters, L., Milner, C. R., Wang, J. X., & Davies, M. J. (2001). Relative risk of conversion from normoglycaemia to impaired glucose tolerance or non-insulin dependent diabetes mellitus in polycystic ovarian syndrome. *Human reproduction, 16*(9), 1995-1998.

[8] Teede, H. J., Hutchison, S., Zoungas, S., & Meyer, C. (2006). Insulin resistance, the metabolic syndrome, diabetes, and cardiovascular disease risk in women with PCOS. *Endocrine, 30*(1), 45-53.

[9] Ataabadi, M. S., Alaee, S., Bagheri, M. J., & Bahmanpoor, S. (2017). Role of Essential Oil of Mentha Spicata (Spearmint) in Addressing Reverse Hormonal and Folliculogenesis Disturbances in a Polycystic Ovarian Syndrome in a Rat Model. *Advanced pharmaceutical bulletin, 7*(4), 651.

[10] Pamela Rackow, Urte Scholz, Rainer Hornung. Received social support and exercising: An

intervention study to test the enabling hypothesis. *British Journal of Health Psychology*, 2015; 20 (4): 763 DOI: 10.1111/bjhp.12139

[11] National Sleep Foundation. *National Sleep Foundation recommends new sleep times.* Retrieved from https://www.sleepfoundation.org/press-release/national-sleep-foundation-recommends-new-sleep-times

[12] American Psychiatric Association. (2013). *Diagnostic and statistical manual of mental disorders (DSM-5®).* American Psychiatric Pub.

www.ingramcontent.com/pod-product-compliance
Lightning Source LLC
Chambersburg PA
CBHW031122250726
48655CB00004B/1806